European School of Oncology

Monographs

Series Editor: U. Veronesi

F. Cavalli (Ed.)

Endocrine Therapy of Breast Cancer

Concepts and Strategies

Springer-Verlag Berlin Heidelberg New York
London Paris Tokyo

Franco Cavalli

Division of Oncology, Ospedale San Giovanni,
6500 Bellinzona, Switzerland

The European School of Oncology gratefully acknowledges sponsorship for the Task Force received from ICI Pharmaceuticals Division, originators and manufacturers of Nolvadex (Trademark).

ISBN-13: 978-3-642-71508-2 e-ISBN-13: 978-3-642-71506-8
DOI: 10.1007/978-3-642-71506-8

Softcover reprint of the hardcover 1st edition 1986

Printing: Beltz Offsetdruck, Hemsbach/Bergstr. Bookbinding: J. Schäffer OHG, Grünstadt
2123/3145-543210

Foreword

Starting in 1986, the European School of Oncology has expanded its activities in postgraduate teaching, which consisted mainly of traditional disease-orientated courses, by promoting new educational initiatives. One of these is the cloister seminars, short meetings intended for highly qualified oncologists and dealing with specific, controversial aspects of clinical practice and research. Another is the institution of permanent study groups, also called task forces, where a limited number of leading experts are invited to meet once a year with the aim of defining the state of the art and possibly reaching a consensus on developments and treatment in specific fields of oncology.

This series of ESO Monographs was designed with the specific purpose of disseminating the results of the most interesting of the seminars and study groups, and providing concise and updated reviews of the subjects discussed.

It was decided to keep the layout very simple in order to keep costs to a minimum and make the monographs available in the shortest possible time, thus overcoming a common problem in medical literature: that of the material being outdated even before publication.

Umberto Veronesi
Chairman, Scientific Committee
European School of Oncology

Table of Contents

How to Read this Monograph

F. Cavalli

Division of Oncology, Ospedale San Giovanni, 6500 Bellinzona, Switzerland

Many potential readers of this book will probably think: "Yet another monograph about breast cancer!". The temptation to rapidly conceal this work in the library, without even an annoyed glance at the table of contents, will therefore be considerable. Are the authors of this monograph the victims of the demands of consumer society, which compel us to the continuous production of books almost nobody will read?

I, personally, do not believe this. But some explanations are certainly needed in order for me to convince the reader to share this belief.

Let us, therefore, first consider the history of this undertaking. It would be more than redundant to elaborate on the increasing role played by the European School of Oncology (ESO). Its courses as well as the recently initiated seminars are already well established. Having set some educational standards for oncology in Europe, the ESO is now extending its work towards research.

As the ancient Greeks already knew, education and research should not be separated. The ESO decided, therefore, to set up a limited number of Task Forces, each encompassing a restricted group of experts (5-8 clinical and basic researchers) who would meet for a 3-day "brain storming" session. Their "only" task would be to establish the state of the art in a certain field of oncology: in doing so, they should mainly concentrate on designing the most important avenues of future research.

The task force on "Endocrine Aspects of Breast Cancer" was the first to meet at Pomerio Castle, Italy, in early April 1986. When we met there we all had the feeling of embarking on a new venture, and we were accordingly very excited. This monograph is the result of our exciting brain storming.

I feel that the authors have, in general, been able to transmit some of this brilliant intellectual enthusiasm to their papers. No, this is not "yet another monograph on breast cancer"!

From the Oncogenes to Some Methodological Questions

The question as to the best therapeutic approach to patients with breast cancer remains a matter of intense debate. This is not only a reflection of continuing clinical controversies, but also of persisting uncertainties at the level of basic research, in spite of a growing collection of experimental data. Our task was to concentrate on the endocrine aspects of breast cancer; however, we did not bypass the results of a wide variety of chemotherapeutic trials. The first three chapters deal basically with experimental strategies for studying the development of breast cancer, with special reference to steroid hormones, growth factors and oncogenes. There is increasing awareness of the close relationship among these entities. The existence of growth factors is really inherent in the concept of hormones, and distinctions between the two may be just semantic. On the other hand, the growth factors, as stressed by Saez, represent a variety of transforming agents or oncogene products in malignant cells. The rapidly growing quantity of data on this topic should be considered with some caution, mainly because of the diversity of the mechnisms involved and of the well-known heterogeneous nature of human breast cancer. Therefore, all three chapters mention different methodological caveats, which will be greatly appreciated by all those actively involved in this exciting line of experimentation.

But the methodological caution should not dampen our intellectual enthusiasm, and the unbiased reader will encounter quite a number of provocative ideas. For instance, I myself am very impressed by the discussion in the chapter by King regarding the central question in breast cancer: How can we explain the transition of a tumour from the hormone-responsive to the unresponsive state? Here are some fundamental statements from his paper: "Thus, oestradiol receptor negative tumours may be of two types, those that have permanently lost their receptors (genotypic-change) and those whose receptor is down-regulated by non-steroidal agents (phenotypic-change). ... The observation that EGF can down-regulate oestradiol and possibly progesterone receptors in cultured breast tumours indicates a mechanism, by which receptor negative cells could be produced." This is a hypothesis put forward by Jordan, who extensively elaborates on it in his comprehensive chapter.

The more clinically oriented chapters are introduced by the contribution by Gelber and Goldhirsch, which I consider to be a milestone in the discussion about the methodology of clinical trials. We all know that clinical trials are fraught with methodological problems and that most controversies stem from suboptimal designs and/or analyses. But only rarely does one find in the literature such a comprehensive and readable presentation of these questions. How many patients do we need in order to observe therapeutic advances in the adjuvant setting? Which are the pitfalls in endocrine trials on advanced breast cancer? What does statistical proof mean? How can we consider a quality of life endpoint in the adjuvant setting? Those, and many others, are the provocative questions raised in this chapter, and I am not going to break the suspense by giving the answers.

Mouridsen gives a careful review of the trials evaluating endocrine treatments for advanced breast cancer and underlines the fact that differences in published results often primarily reflect differences in patient selection. He also raises the problem of the best sequence of endocrine treatments in postmenopausal patients. This question is of utmost importance since we, and others, have recently demonstrated that in most postmenopausal women with advanced breast cancer, hormone therapy remains the first-choice treatment (1-3). Goldhirsch, Gelber and Mouridsen then discuss the results of some of the most important trials in the adjuvant setting. Particular attention is devoted to the relative merits of endocrine treatment and of the combination of chemotherapy and hormone treatment. This aspect is re-emphasized in the somewhat more speculative contribution by Jordan, dealing with the possible optimal strategy for adjuvant therapy of breast cancer. Of special interest here is the discussion concerning the prolonged use of tamoxifen in postmenopausal women as well as the still poorly understood role of this antioestrogen in premenopausal women. Tamoxifen therapy in premenopausal patients may not be an optimal long-term strategy, as increased steroidogenesis may ultimately cause tumour regrowth. This raises the question of performing concomitant oophorectomy in order to create a low oestrogen environment.

Since we still do not know the possible impact of many years of tamoxifen treatment on the endocrine system of premenopausal women, Jordan underlines in his conclusive chapter the great caution with which prophylactic trials with this drug should be managed, stating that they should only be undertaken in "normal high-risk premenopausal women."

What Next ?

These are only some of the highlights of this monograph and I am sure that the readers will discover many others. And we intend to pursue our efforts. We shall meet again in the spring of 1987. In the meantime new data will have accumulated. Possibly some of the provocative hypotheses will already have been translated into experimental data. In addition, we shall concentrate on some other topics, which were only briefly touched upon in this first monograph. We shall then concentrate on the whole area of markers, including the clinical importance of receptors, which we were not able to fully cover this time. And we have already decided to focus on another important methodological problem: Are our current methods and means of measuring tumour response really adaquate? Or should we rather look for a more appropriate methodology in the objective assessment of clinical trials?

There can be no doubt that in one year you can look forward to the next issue: another provocative monograph.

Acknowledgements

In the name of all authors of this monograph I would like to acknowledge the excellent help of the staff of the European School of Oncology (ESO) in arranging the meeting at Pomerio Castle as well as in preparing this monograph.
In particular, we also thank ICI for the generous grant which made this undertaking possible.

References

1. Cavalli F, Beer M, Martz G et al: Concurrent or sequential use of cytotoxic chemotherapy and hormone treatment in advanced breast cancer. Report of the Swiss Group for Clinical Cancer Research. Br Med J 1983 (286): 5-8
2. Australian and New Zealand Breast Cancer Trials Group, Clinical Oncological Society of Australia. A randomized trial in postmenopausal patients with advanced breast cancer comparing endocrine and cytotoxic therapy given sequentially or in combination. J Clin Oncol 1986 (4): 186-193
3. Taylor SG, Gelman RS, Folkson G et al: Combination chemotherapy compared to tamoxifen as initial therapy for stage IV breast cancer in elderly women. Ann Int Med 1986 (104):455-461

Experimental Strategies for Studying the Development of Breast Cancer with Special Reference to Steroid Hormones, Growth Factors and Oncogenes

R.J.B. King

Hormone Biochemistry Department, Imperial Cancer Research Fund, P.O. Box 123, Lincoln's Inn Fields, London WC2A 3PX, UK

I INTRODUCTION

The growth factor revolution has arrived and it can safely be predicted that an enormous literature will be generated on its application to hormone sensitive tumours such as breast cancer. Some of that literature will be even useful. It is universally agreed that breast cancer is a multifaceted disease and yet it is not always clear which feature is being addressed in some of the current research. This paper will attempt to highlight what I think are the important biological features of breast cancer that should be considered both in the design and interpretation of experiments in this area. Attention will be confined to the interrelationships of steroid hormones and their non-steroidal counterparts with oncogenes and growth factors. Because experiences of the latter components have developed from cell and molecular biological experimentation, it is not surprising that much of the current application to breast neoplasia should be via the same methods. In particular, the use of cell lines in culture is almost mandatory for many of the experiments because of their simplicity relative to whole animal or clinical studies. Due to the paucity of cell lines that are steroid sensitive, this approach has of necessity been directed at the regulation of established tumour cells. However, it should not be assumed that data so derived will also apply to other components of neoplasia such as initiation, progression, invasion or metastasis. What is clear is that information generated from the use of tumour cell lines should be used as a basis for studies on these and other aspects, to see if there is any common ground. This theme will be adopted for the present article. I will not attempt to encompass all the somewhat fragmentary data currently available but will develop ideas based on a more general approach and will attempt to highlight what I think are areas of biology that deserve attention.

II GENERAL ASPECTS OF ONCOGENE AND GROWTH FACTOR RESEARCH

Ideas about oncogenes and protooncogenes have been around in one form or another for a long time but came to fruition with the molecular dissection of oncogenic viruses (for general reviews consult references 4,5,7 and 8). This showed that oncogenic retroviruses (RNA viruses capable of producing DNA copies that stably integrate into host DNA) have acquired, during their evolution, DNA sequences from host cells and that these sequences are vital for the neoplastic potential of the virus. These viral sequences or oncogenes (v-onc) are, therefore, also present in normal, uninfected cells albeit in somewhat different forms, the so-called proto-or cellular oncogenes (c-onc). A given c-onc can be modified in several ways by different viruses as for example has occurred with the v-ras family.

Modified c-oncs do not transform cells by a common pathway (see below). They can broadly be divided into two classes depending on whether they immortalize cells (Class 1) or diminish anchorage dependence (Class 2).
Products of the former are predominantly nuclear and the latter extranuclear. More is known about the extranuclear proteins. They can be either growth factors (e.g. sis), analogues of growth factor receptors (e.g. erb-B) or agents that transduce the signal generated by the receptor (e.g. ras). The existence of these multiple pathways should be borne in mind when applying data derived from breast tumour cell lines to normal or hyperplastic cells, as for example will be necessary for studies on carcinogenesis.

Furthermore, not all transforming viruses express oncogenes: mouse mammary tumour virus (MMTV) is a case in point. Its intimate involvement in murine mammary tumorigenesis seems to be due to the insertion of regulatory elements adjacent to certain cellular structural genes. The cellular gene involved is different in different strains of mice. Additionally, in some strains of mice a putative oncogene (orf) is transcribed from the long terminal repeat of the virus.

The diversity of mechanisms inherent in these data, together with the heterogeneous nature of human breast cancer, should be borne in mind in considering experiments on breast cancer but should not dampen enthusiasm for this line of experimentation.

A major advance occurred with the advent of transfection experiments in which cellular transforming DNA is introduced into cultured cells and their phenotype changed from the normal to the transformed state. This enables the identification of transforming genes and thereby widens the scope of the oncogene model to non-virally infected cells. However, the majority of transforming genes so far identified turned out to be analogues of v-oncs. All the initial transection experiments utilized cell lines as the recipient cells and single genes were identified that could induce transformation. This may be surprising when one considers evidence from epidemiological and other sources that multiple genetic changes must be involved in tumour development (34). The anomaly is partly resolved by the fact that cultured cell lines are not normal but have been immortalized by selective pressure in culture; genetic changes have occurred to enable their long-term survival in culture. Recognition of this fact has led to information on the cooperation of multiple oncogenes and it has been possible to allocate oncogenes to one of two classes depending on whether they immortalize cells but do not induce full neoplasia (Class 1) or produce fully transformed cells from immortalized cells (Class 2) (67).

Virtually all of the culture work with human breast cancer has been performed with cell lines derived from pleural effusion.

Such metastatic cells may have progressed a long way from the initial neoplastic events even prior to selection in culture. Such considerations should not detract from their continued use only to exhort caution in widening the application of data so derived to other situations.

The existence of growth factors is really inherent in the concept of hormones and, in the present climate, distinction between the two may be semantic. However, I will use both terms with hormones referring to the classic, blood-borne, factors and growth factors referring to the more recent protein/peptide components that tend to act at a more local level. (For general reviews on growth factors consult references 19,46,61.)

The impact of growth factors on thinking related to tumorigenesis stems from two observations. First are the data showing that cells can secrete products that regulate either their own function (autocrine) or those of nearby cells of a different type (paracrine) (58). Second are the observations that link the function of putative v-oncs to the actions of growth factors: the v-sis product with platelet derived growth factor (PDGF), v-erb B with epidermal growth factor (EGF) receptor and v-fms colony stimulating factor (19). More recently this speculation has been extended to homologies between steroid receptors and another viral product of unknown function, v-erb A (20,21,68).

Most discussions of the general points made above imply stimulation of processes involved in growth regulation; it is important to remember that regulation can also be disrupted by switching off cell functions. Genetic evidence from tumours like Wilms and retinoblastoma (57) and cell experis between normal and tumour cells (52) point to the involvement of recessive rather than dominant features in at least some cancers.

III CELL BIOLOGY OF CULTURED BREAST CANCER CELLS

Virtually all of the data contained in the preceding section were derived from culture experiments with cell lines. In relating the hypotheses contained therein to their potential impact on the many facets of breast cancer, a logical starting point is hormone-sensitive, breast cancer cell lines. (For reviews, consult references 28,35,56,71). It is also reasonable to consider cell proliferation as an important index of that sensitivity. The growth pattern of two such cell lines are shown in Figs. 1 (S115 androgen responsive mouse mammary tumour cell line) and 2 (ZR-75-1 oestrogen responsive human mammary tumour cell line).

Despite the fact that one line is of murine origin and responds to androgen (Fig. 1), whilst the other is derived from a human breast pleural effusion and responds to oestrogen (Fig. 2), three general points can be made that relate to the topic of oncogenes and growth factors (Table 1).

Growth occurs in the absence of steroid which indicates that they are not essential for this cell function. This simplistic but important statement carries implications for various aspects of

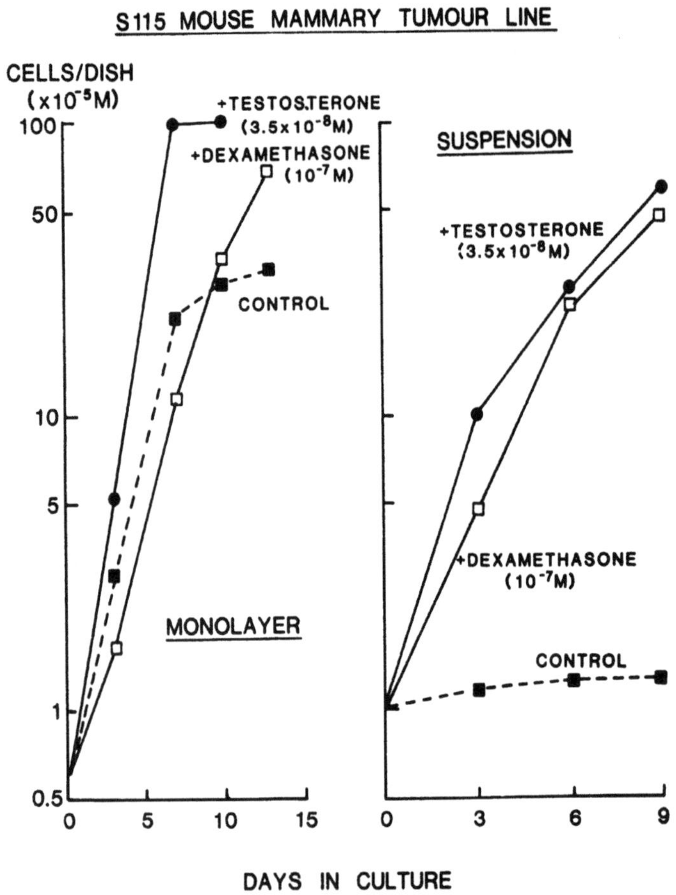

Figure 1. Sensitivity of S115 mouse mammary tumour cell line to steroids under different growth conditions. All cultures contained 5% charcoal-stripped, foetal calf serum.

tumour development that will be referred to in section VI. The caveat that must be applied to conclusions from this type of experiment is that the culture medium contains serum. Despite removal of free steroids with dextran charcoal, one cannot be certain that all metabolites capable of conversion to active components have been so removed. It is therefore important that serum-free media be developed capable of long-term maintenance of such cells in steroid-sensitive states. Such media will also be essential for studies on the interaction of steroids and growth factors, as serum is a mixture of such factors and it is already known that complex interactions occur between growth factors. All of the essential features listed in Table 1 can be produced in serum-free conditions, at least with the human cells (9). It should also be remembered that some breast tumour cells can make their own oestrogen although that is not the case with ZR-75-1 cells (44).

In monolayer culture, cells attach to the plastic substrate and at low density proliferation is accelerated by androgen (S115 cells) (71) or oestrogen (ZR-75-1 cells) (11) and inhibited by glucocorticoids (both cell lines). This log phase or exponential growth of cells is the feature most commonly referred to in publications although linear growth curves are often presented which indicates abnormal behaviour for cells that are supposed to multiply in a logarithmic fashion. Although hormonal effects on logarithmic growth are real they are not large with maximum three-fold changes in growth rate being obtained. On the other hand, large and different steroid responses are observed with less frequently reported features of cell behaviour like saturation density and suspension growth. Both these properties

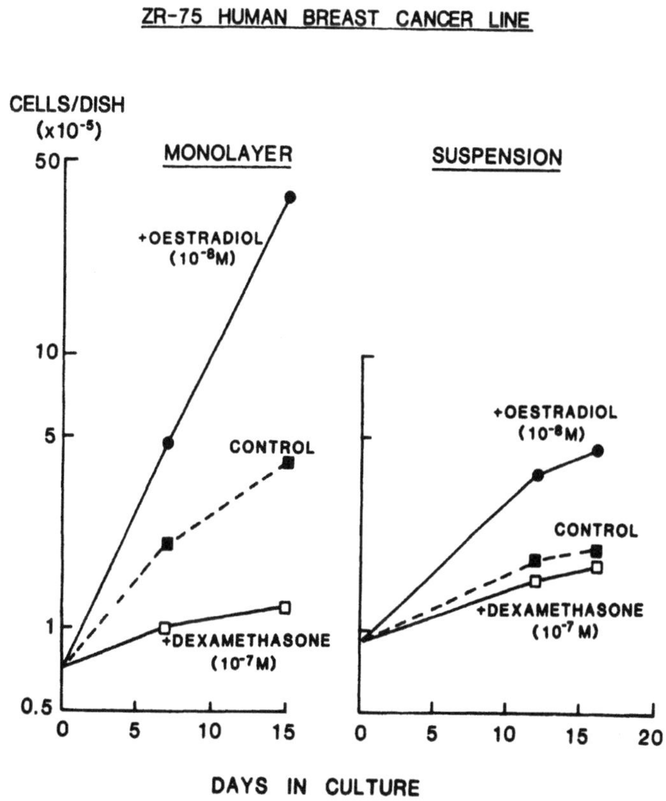

Fig. 2. Sensitivity of ZR-75-1 human mammary tumour cell line to steroids under different growth conditions. All cultures contained 5% charcoal-stripped, foetal calf serum.

Table 1

Steroid sensitivities of cultured breast tumour cell lines

1. Cells grow in absence of steroid
2. Steroids affect at least four properties (log-phase growth, saturation density, suspension growth, morphology (data not shown)
3. Each of these properties can be modulated independently by suitable choice of steroid and growth conditions

are stimulated by androgen/oestrogen, whereas glucocorticoid effects depend on the cell line. Suspension growth is stimulated in mouse cells and inhibited in the human line. The ability to grow both to higher densities in monolayer culture and without attachment to the substrate (suspension or anchorage independence) reflect major changes in the ability of cells to recognise their environment. Another example of the way the external environment can influence cell function comes from the observation that oestradiol induction of progesterone receptor occurs when normal mammary cells are plated on either an inert matrix or dead cells, but that a substrate of live cells is necessary for oestradiol stimulation of DNA synthesis (24). The molecular signals required for these other features are not necessarily identical to those required for log phase growth (42). In the present context, it is important to note that one of the standard methods for detecting and assaying transforming growth factors is their ability to promote anchorage independent growth. Clearly this feature of steroid mediated cell function is a prime candidate for studies on growth factors.

Morphological changes in both cell lines accompany these changes in behaviour. With the mouse cells in monolayer culture, these are evident under the light microscope as a transition from epithelial to fibroblastic shape (72), whereas more subtle changes occur with the human cells and electron microscopic observations are required (65). These observations are important because of the influence cell shape has on proliferation rates (42).

The general features described in this section and summarised in Table 1 carry important messages both for the design and interpretation of experiments aimed at elucidating the role of growth factors/oncogenes in steroid mediated cell growth in culture. Firstly, attention should not be confined to only one behavioural feature such as log-phase growth as in this way other, possibly more important changes will be missed. Secondly, it should be made clear what feature is actually being studied. Unfortunately, this apparently obvious statement is not always observed. Thirdly, the molecular changes accompanying one cell feature will not necessarily be the same as those associated with a different feature. Therefore it is important to relate biochemistry to a particular cell function, otherwise confusion will be generated in the literature because of not comparing like with like. I am, however, rather sanguine about compliance with this request. Finally, it is apparent that by judicious choice of culture conditions and steroid, the main features of cell behaviour and the molecular events that mediate them can be dissected.

All such studies of biochemistry and behaviour are of necessity correlative and, whilst giving strong indications of the importance or otherwise of a given pathway, do not provide absolute proof. There is a pressing need for the generation of cell variants, particularly of the temperature-sensitive type, in order to provide that proof; no mutant cell lines exist that are temperature-sensitive for steroid-mediated cell changes.

Also required are experimental systems for analysing the transition from hormone-sensitive to insensitive state. Serial transplantation or growth *in vivo* interspersed with periods in culture (6,27) have been productive in delineating pathways of progression and have shown that cell selection is important. However, these methods cannot define the molecular events involved in the initial change in sensitivity. Cell culture systems would help in this area. Mutagens have been used to generate hormone insensitive lymphoma cell lines (54) but it is not known if the same mechanism applies to breast cancer. The S115 mouse mammary tumour cell line spontaneously becomes hormone (androgen) insensitive when deprived of androgen and some of the molecular events have been dissected (10). Other systems of this type are required.

It is far from clear as to how these cell biological events relate to *in vivo* behaviour. Clearly changes in proliferation rate are important but what about the other changes discussed here? Are they related to changes in tumour size or to other properties such as invasion or metastases? These important, unanswered questions should be addressed. They are discussed further in section V.

IV BIOCHEMICAL RESPONSES OF CULTURED BREAST CELLS

For reviews consult references 36, 48, 55.
The present picture is adequately but incompletely described by the model shown in Fig. 3. Under physiological conditions there is little, if any, firm evidence for non-receptor mediated pathways being important. At the pharmacological level, which is clearly important in the context of cancer treatment, the situation is less clear-cut. Antioestrogens have two major effects on cultured breast cells.

Growth is inhibited (cytostatic effect) at modest concentrations ($< 10^{-6}$M) whilst the cells are killed at high concentrations (cytocidal effect); the former is receptor mediated, the latter is not, although antioestrogen binding sites may be involved (45, 63). Discussion centres on what is the biologically effective *in-vivo* concentration of tamoxifen?
The evidence favours the cytotoxic effects as being the more important.

Pathways of response can be divided into the three routes (Fig. 3). At the present time it is impossible to comment on the relative importance of each of these pathways and it is likely that all three routes are utilised, possibly to different degrees in different tumours. Route 1 involves direct stimulation of the proliferation pathways. Whilst DNA polymerase and nucleotide pools are increased by steroid hormones at the start of S phase of the cell cycle, these are relatively late effects of the hormone. Alterations in non-histone chromosomal proteins and enzymes like creatine kinase BB are potential candidates but most current interest centres on routes 2 and 3. In fact the distinction between these two pathways may be semantic. There is no doubt that steroids do change the proliferative sensitivity of cells to growth factors in serum (11) but it is not known if this is via routes 2 or 3. Also, not represented in Fig. 3 are the da-

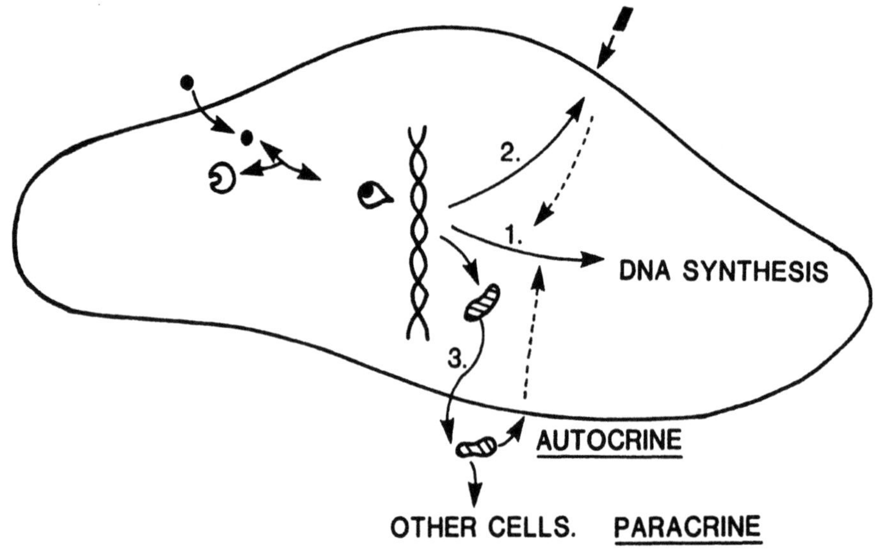

1. DIRECT ACTION
2. CHANGE MEMBRANE SENSITIVITY TO EXTERNAL STIMULI (CELLS/GROWTH FACTORS)
3. PRODUCE GROWTH FACTORS

Figure 3. Potential routes by which steroids (•) can influence cell proliferation. native receptor; activated steroid receptor complex; chromatin

ta indicating steroid effects on more remote cells which can make regulatory molecules such as the estromedins (55). Actions of such blood-borne growth factors could be allocated to route 2.

Steroid effects described in section III on the way that mammary tumour cells interact with their environment implies important multiple changes in membrane receptors. Thus far, attention has been limited to a few such receptors but a broadening of this approach will be rewarding. Understandably, EGF receptor has dominated the literature thus far but membrane receptors for other growth factors, cells or extracellular matrix components will yield interesting data. It is already clear from the EGF receptor data that such experiments will have to be carefully performed and cautiously interpreted. Experiments using radiolabelled EGF to assay receptor levels have shown that receptor number can be regulated by steroid hormones in some cases. However, in some cells (uterus) oestrogen is the agonist (40) whilst in others progestins (39) are the stimulant (breast cancer cells). Furthermore there is no obvious correlation between receptor number and responsiveness to EGF (16). The reason for changes in EGF binding must be determined as multiple mechanisms exist. Receptor occupancy by ligand results in internalisation which may be accompanied by recycling of the receptor but not the ligand. Analysis of both membranes and intact cells will be required to dissect these pathways and binding studies should be complemented by experiments with both immunological and nucleic acid probes, all of which are now available. The affinity of RGF receptor for EGF can be decreased

by other growth factors without changing receptor number (49, 73). Finally, with the v-erb B data in mind, one must recognise the possibility that breast cells may have functional EGF receptor in the absence of a ligand binding site.
There is unequivocal evidence that both autocrine and paracrine effects are important (route 3). Cultured breast cancer cells secrete PDGF which is known to influence both stromal and endothelial cell proliferation (51). Also, human breast cancer cells have greater angiogenic potential than normal epithelium (23) (paracrine effects). The existence of autocrine pathways has been known for some time and considerable attention is now being directed at the characterisation of those factors. Several have been identified in biological fluids such as milk (74) and breast cyst fluid (22) and in medium from cultured cells (13, 31, 36, 48, 75). Special attention is being focused on transforming growth factors(s) (α TGF) which are secreted in an oestrogen-responsive manner by mammary tumour cells (13,36). TGFs are a group of polypeptides related to EGF which apparently function by binding to the EGF receptor (47, 61). It has been suggested that they are embryonic forms of EGF (61). Several different, but related TGFs have been identified but it is not clear if they are all physiologically relevant or whether some represent metabolites or methodological artefacts.

It is already clear that α TGFs/EGF are important in the biology of breast cancer but it is probable that other growth factors are also involved. It should be recalled that experiments to define serum-free media for breast cells highlighted the absolute requirement for transferrin (3) and that the number of membrane transferrin receptors can reflect the proliferative state of cells. The basis for these over-dogmatic statements about EGF is as follows: EGF stimulates proliferation of some breast cells, (16,37,60), EGF/TGFs have been identified as breast-related (see above) products and the known actions of these factors can explain some of the steroid-mediated responses of breast tumour cells (see section III).

A link between these growth factors and oncogenes has not been established for breast cancer cells. Hormone effects on oncogene expression in cultured mammary tumour cells are currently being studied but here are too few data to warrant comment other than to say that several analogues of the viral oncogenes are expressed.

V IN-VIVO EFFECTS OF STEROID HORMONES

For general reviews on this topic, see other chapters in this monograph and references 50 and 69.
How do the cell biological changes relate to in-vivo responses? The plain answer is that we do not know. No one would doubt that changes in growth rate have important consequences in-vivo but it is more difficult to relate changes in saturation density, serum requirements or anchorage independence to in-vivo events. Given the practical importance of the questions being posed, it is essential to identify the in-vivo and cell culture correlates. For example, the work on EGF/TGF has raised both speculation and

financial input into its therapeutic applications. We know that a major effect of these growth factors is to promote anchorage independence. If we do not know the clinical consequences of such changes, it is difficult to decide which aspect of treatment would be most rewarding. Obviously, lack of such correlates should not stop developmental work but, through ignorance, it might limit the applications of such work. It is my feeling that information from the cell culture experiments is providing the clues as to which parameters are worth studying with clinical material and from this we will acquire the correlative information required.
This section will deal with certain aspects of that process in relation to the growth factor model.

Fig. 4 illustrates a widely held view of neoplastic progression as it applies to both human breast and endometrium. Why bring endometrium into discussions of breast cancer? I am convinced that studies on hormonal events in endometrium can provide complementary and, in some cases, unique data that cannot be obtained with breast. For example, normal endometrium is readily available but the same cannot be said for breast. Furthermore, animal data suggest that the hormonal requirements of endometrium are less complex than those of breast in the sense that pituitary hormones like prolactin do not confuse interpretation of in-vivo experiments. Finally, the risk factors common to both breast and endometrial cancer indicate that at least some of the features of the two diseases are similar. I would agree, however, with critics of this approach, that important differences between breast and endometrium do exist and that results from endometrium must not be applied in an uncritical manner to breast. Differences in hormonal effects on cell proliferation (1,33), on pituitary hormone requirements and in tumour incidence consequent to hormone replacement therapy (oestrogen) (64) attest to that fact.

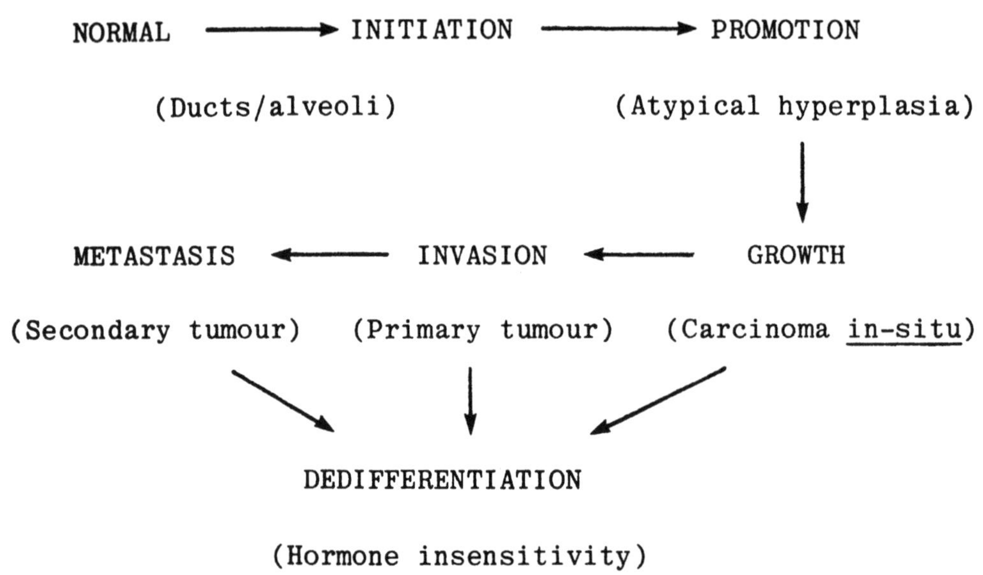

Figure 4. Putative pathway of carcinogenesis and tumour progression with tissues that may represent a given stage of that pathway.

Table 2

AVAILABILITY OF HUMAN TISSUES

	BREAST	ENDOMETRIUM
Normal	+	++
Benign Hyperplasia	+	+
Atypical Hyperplasia	±	±
Carcinoma in-situ	+	±
Primary Tumour	++	+
Secondary Tumour	+	+
Hormone Responsive Tumour	+	+
Hormone Unresponsive Tumour	+	+

Steroids could influence each and every stage illustated in Fig. 4 so how can they be studied? Also shown in Fig. 4 are tissues that could provide information about that stage of progression whilst Table 2 lists the availability of those tissues. I am well aware that there are defects in my identification of certain pathological entities as being representative of a given stage of progression.

Criticism is most justified for the association of atypical hyperplasia with promotion. I have two reasons, one scientific and the other pragmatic, for making that association. I am impressed by the results with both breast (14,43) and endometrium (29), indicating the degree to which atypical hyperplasias are associated with either subsequent or concurrent cancer. This does not prove its direct involvement in progression but I consider it to be the best available material for studying this important phase of carcinogenesis.
I would also apply this logic to the other allocations of tissues to stage of progression shown in Fig. 4.

Some comment is required about the availabilities of tissues listed in Table 2. Disturbingly little is known about the hormonal regulation of normal human breast epithelium. The obvious choice is tissue from premenopausal women whose use of contraceptive agents, parity and stage of menstrual cycle is known. Material is occasionally available from reduction mammoplasties but a more abundant sous normal breast adjacent to fibroadenomas removed at surgery. Although the number of such samples can be high, the amount of tissue per sample is small, which will dictate the analytical methods that can be used. Autoradiographic analysis of DNA synthesis is proving useful but the increasing availability of immunological and c'DNA probes for oncogenes and their products and for growth factors should make histochemical approaches rewarding. The same can be said for the hyperplasias and carcinoma <u>in-situ</u> which are most frequently encountered in association with invasive cancer. The potential rewards of such approaches can be judged by reference to histochemical data on an antigen that is qualitatively and quantitatively related to ER (30) (Fig. 5). The antigen is low in normal human mammary epithelium and high in most ER positive tumours; carcinoma in-situ seems to be the intermediate stage both in terms of staining intensity and heterogeneity. Other examples of increased antigen accumulation in tumour as compared to normal mammary epithelium can be cited and it is clearly of importance to identify the pathological stages at which the changes occur.

At present, the ability to characterise the hormone sensitivity of a given tumour relies on steroid receptor analysis. Their defects for this purpose are well-known but are not sufficient to detract from use; molecular differences between receptor negative and receptor positive samples would be expected on some but not all occasions.

What should be assayed? In our present level of ignorance it would be not a bad approach to screen all available reagents related to oncogenes and growth factors, but for laboratories without such facilities, there are some hints as to which might be the more fruitful avenues. Cell culture experiments have indicated the importance of EGF/ αTGF whilst ER negative tumours tend to have higher levels of EGF receptor than their ER positive counterparts (15,53), so these components warrant attention. The interrelationship between receptors for steroids and growth factors are discussed in section VI and in the articles by Jordan and Saez in this monograph. All that will be said at this point is that, given the complexities of receptor numerology (section II), the physiological significance of these observations remains to be established. If one assumes that elevated EGF receptor represents increased output of or sensitivity to TGF, what is it telling us?
Are such cells growing more rapidly or is the shorter disease-free interval a reflection of a greater metastatic potential? As pointed out in section III, a major effect of TGF is the promotion of anchorage independent growth which, in the case of breast tumour cell lines, means growing as discrete clumps of cells. Experimental work with melanoma has indicated that cell clumps are more likely to metastases than individual cells. Speculations of this type may be wrong, but it would be equally wrong to interpret all effects as being due to alterations in proliferation rate.

Likewise, one could speculate on the basis for the high amounts of elastic tissue in tumours having a favourable prognosis. Could this, together with abnormal behaviour of fibroblasts from breast cancer patients (2), be due to PDGF secretion?

Turning to oncogenes, one can construct at least one tenable hypothesis capable of experimental testing. Dogma states that oestrogens are promotors rather than initiators (8,29). As a generalization, this is probably correct although it is evident from Fig. 4 that there are other important loci that could be, and probably are, influenced by steroids. However, if one assumes dogma to be correct, what predictions could be made about oncogene expression? As stated earlier (section II) oncogenes can

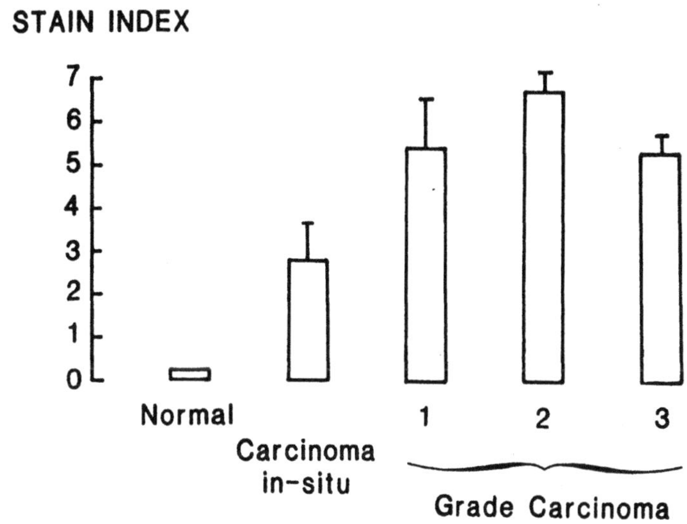

Figure 5. Histochemical analysis of an oestrogen-receptor related protein (P29) in ductal epithelia of human breast.

broadly be classified according to whether they immortalize cells (Class 1) or promote anchorage independence (Class 2). Could it be that immortalization is equivalent to initiation and progression to anchorage independence? A consequence of such speculation would be that certain Class 2 oncogenes should be hormone-sensitive. Selective data can be quoted in support of the idea. Anchorage independence is the best, albeit incomplete, cell biological correlate of tumour promotion and steroids certainly promote that independence (section III). It may not be chance that ras oncogene (a member of Class 2) products are hormone-sensitive in DMBA-induced rat mammary tumours (12), have prognostic significance in human prostatic cancer (66), and that the ras gene is changed in chemically-induced rat mammary tumours (62). An important publication from both the conceptual and methodological point of view, describes the development of mammary tumours in transgenic mice (59). The myc oncogene (Class 1) was coupled to a viral promoter, inserted into fertilised eggs which were then implanted into pseudopregnant mice. Some of the progeny had a high incidence of pregnancy-dependent tumours. The authors suggest that myc expression is necessary but insufficient for tumour development and that additional hormone-sensitive events are involved.

Too much should not be made of these rather wild speculations based on two very broad generalizations but I do feel that the idea of looking at combinations of certain oncogenes from the two general classes at different stages of tumour progression will be worthwhile.

VI HORMONE INSENSITIVITY

If one accepts, as I do, that some of the hormone effects on breast cancer are mediated by growth factors or related products, what consequences follow concerning the transition from hormone responsive to unresponsive state? The simplest hypothesis would be that in the unresponsive tumour, production of or sensitivity to growth factors has escaped from hormonal control. A plausible variant of that model is that different growth factors or pathways of response become operative. Transfection of MCF-7 human breast cancer cell line with a ras oncogene results in hormosensitive growth (26,36). The ras product is thought to act by transducing membrane signals to the interior of the cell so this could be cited in support of the model. The growth factor model has important implications for the long held concept that loss of steroid receptor activity is a central event in the transition to insensitivity.
To me, it implies the opposite, namely that loss of steroid receptor is a consequence rather than a cause of insensitivity.

Evidence for loss of receptor activity being central to loss of sensitivity comes mainly from two sources. Firstly, steroid responsive normal cells have receptors whilst unresponsive normal cells do not (32). When tested with tumours, the same general pattern was observed but there were an appreciable number of exceptions in which receptors were present but the tumour was insensitive (25). The idea of post-receptor defects was developed to explain such tumours. Secondly, the pioneering work on glucocorticoid sensitivity of lymphoma variants indicated that the majority of insensitive variants had lost receptor activity (54). Recent work with receptor antibodies suggests that the whole receptor and not just the ligand binding site is lost (38, 41, 70). Of the receptor positive but insensitive variants, most had an abnormal receptor machinery whilst post-receptor defects were invoked to explain the remaining phenotype.

In the light of more recent results, the relevance of these two sets of data to tumours stimulated by hormones can be questioned.

The model in Fig. 6 outlines the basis for my thoughts in this area. If one adopts the view that steroid receptor activity is the prime requisite for growth regulation and that regulation is mediated by growth factors, it is difficult to immediately reconcile loss of receptor activity with increased growth factor production. One possible explanation would be that loss of steroid binding site is not accompanied by loss of the functional part of the receptor and that this modified receptor is active in the absence of ligand. However, this very reasonable idea is receiving little support from the immunoassay data on either breast tumours or experimental lymphomas; the predicted appearance of a substantial number of ligand binding negative, antibody-positive tumours has not happened. This may reflect the limited number of antibodies thus far used, but I doubt it. A second possibility, not shown in Fig. 6, is that the steroid is switching off an inhibitor analogous to a chalone. However, loss of receptor activity would result in constitutive levels of inhibitor.

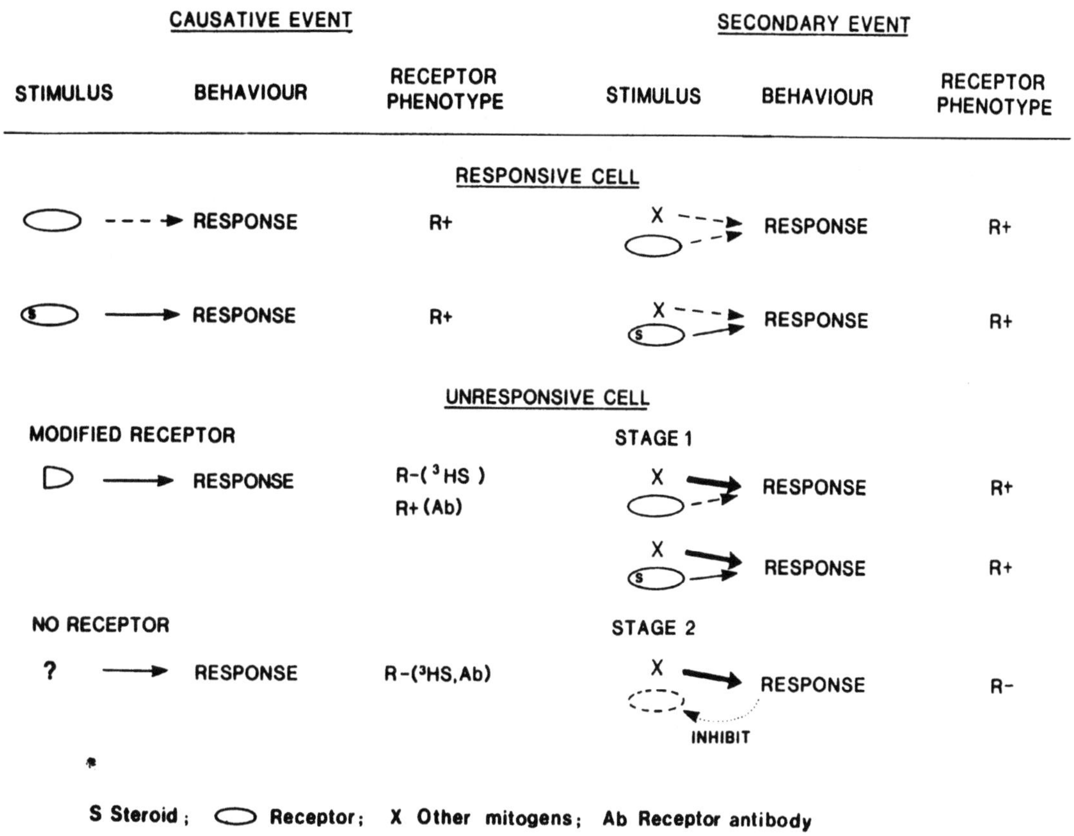

Figure 6. Unresponsive breast tumours: are changes in steroid receptor a cause of insensitivity or secondary to other changes?

This alone would not explain the data and one would have to further speculate that the inhibitor is in turn blocking a pathway that negatively affects cell function. Whilst not ruling out such a double negative pathway, I do not find it attractive.

Events that better describe the biologial behaviour of breast tumour cells are presented in the right-hand side of Fig. 6. The basic premise, amply substantiated by experimental evidence, is that steroids are only one of many sets of reagents that influence growth (section III). The responsive state is depicted as a balance between steroid-mediated and X-mediated (growth factor?) events. In Fig. 6, steroid and mitogen are shown feeding into a common pathway (route 2, Fig. 3) but it could be readily adapted to an autocrine mechanism in which steroid increases the concentration of mitogen (route 3, Fig. 3). The unresponsive state might result from increased mitogenic activity through no influence of steroid. The steroid pathway could be fully functional but its effects swamped by the other pathway; a receptor positive but unresponsive tumour. Prolonged production of mitogen, by making the receptor mechanism redundant, could eventually result in the production of receptor negative cells. Thus, oestradiol receptor negative tumours may be of two types, those that have permanently lost their receptors (genotypic change) and those whose receptor is down-regulated by non-steroidal agents (phenotypic change). It may be possible to restore the phenotype of the latter category and thus restore hormone sensitivity. The observation that EGF can down-regulate oestradiol (Jordan, this monograph) and possibly progesterone (49) receptors in cultured breast tumours indicates a mechanism by which receptor negative cells could be produced.

The hypothesis presented in Fig. 6 is speculative, but I find it easier to accommodate the current data on hormone unresponsive tumours with the idea that loss of steroid receptor is a consequence rather than a cause of hormone insensitivity. I see no conflict with the two original premises on which the original model was based (see above). The presence or absence of steroid receptors in normal cells is a true reflecton of their function and is not relevant to the very different situation in which responsive tumour cells change to an unresponsive state. The lymphoma data can be questioned on its relevance to breast cancer. Glucocorticoids kill responsive lumphoma cells by a different mechanism to that by which oestrogens stimulate breast proliferation. Loss of receptor probably is the prime reason for resistance to killing in lymphoma; I see no basis for automatically transposing that model to the stimulatory situation seen with breast cancer.

Whether or not steroid receptor changes are a consequence or cause of unresponsiveness is not simply an academic exercise. The idea of reverting an unresponsive tumour to the responsive state has often been raised because of the beneficial clinical consequences. If receptor loss is consequent to the other changes, then modulation of those changes might restore endocrine sensitivity. For example, if α TGF production is increased in receptor positive, unresponsive breast tumours, its suppression in addition to being desirable in its own right, might make the tumour amenable to hormone therapy.

A second sequel of the cause or consequence discussion concerns the considerable effort currently devoted to the identification of postreceptor defects in receptor positive but unresponsive breast tumours. The consequence model would indicate that such studies may not be productive.

The points raised in this section are largely hypothetical and have been presented as ideas that may provoke novel avenues of research. I do favour the consequence model and its sequellae but I would not reject the idea of some tumours having postreceptor defects which render them hormone insensitive. My long involvement in breast cancer research has taught me not to expect any one model to provoke the absolute truth!

FUTURE WORK

Based on the ideas promoted in this article, I would suggest the following aspects to be of prime importance. They are all amenable to experimentation.

Methodology

1. The generation of more hormone-sensitive cell lines from both normal and neoplastic breast. The limited number of tumour lines means that we are uncertain as to how typical their responses are. Also, the dearth of lines from normal epithelium prevents comparison between normal and neoplastic breast. The apparent contradiction in terms of having a normal cell line should not inhibit this development.

2. Long term serum-free culture. It will not be possible to test some of the hypotheses on autocrine and paracrine regulation without these methods.

3. Generation of variants that are insensitive to steroids; temperature-sensitive mutants would be the most rewarding. I see this as being the single most important methodological advance that can be made. Without such mutants, absolute proof of direct relationships between a given parameter and steroid sensitivity cannot be established.

Conceptual approaches

1. Interaction of cultured normal and tumour cells with their environment.

2. Relevance of cell biological characteristics to in-vivo and clinical behaviour.

3. Analysis of normal, hyperplastic and neoplastic human breast with immunological and nucleic acid probes.

4. Interrelationships between growth factors and receptors with respect to hormone sensitivity.

ACKNOWLEDGEMENTS

I am indebted to Philippa Darbre for allowing the presentation of her data on steroid sensitivity of cultured cell lines and to the many staff members of the Imperial Cancer Research Fund who have helped in the development of ideas presented here.

REFERENCES

1. Anderson TJ, Ferguson DJP and Raab GM: Cell turnover in the resting human breast: influence of parity, contraceptive pill, age and laterality. Br J Cancer 1982 (46):376-382
2. Azzarone B, Mareel M, Billard C, Scemama P, Chaponmnier C and Macieira-Coelho A: Abnormal properties of skin fibroblasts from patients with breast cancer. Int J Cancer 1984 (33):759-764
3. Barnes D and Stato G: Growth of human mammary tumour cell line in a serum-free medium. Nature 1979 (281):388-389

4. Bishop JM: Viral oncogenes. Cell 1985 (42):23-38
5. Bishop JM: Oncogenes. Scientific American 1982 (246):68-79
6. Bruchovsky N and Rennie PS: Classification of dependent and autonomous variants of Shionogi mammary carcinoma based on heterogeneous patterns of androgen binding. Cell 1978 (13):273-280
7. Cooper GM: Activation of cellular transforming genes in neoplasms. In: Bresciani F, King RJB, Lippman ME, Raynaud JP and Namer M (eds): Hormone and cancer progress in cancer research and therapy 1983 (31):1-6 New York: Raven Press
8. Day NE: Epidemiological evidence of promoting effects - the example of breast cancer. In: Hecker E, Fusening NE, Kunz W, Marks F and Theilmann HW (eds): Carcinogenesis 1982 (7):183-199 New York: Raven Press
9. Darbre PD, Curtis S and King RJB: Effects of estradiol and tamoxifen on human breast cells in serum-free culture. Cancer Res 1984 (44):2790-2793
10. Darbre P and King RJB: Progression to steroid autonomy in S115 mouse mammary tumor cells: role of DNA methylation. J Cell Biol 1984 (99):1410-1415
11. Darbre P, Yates J, Curtis and King RJB: Effect of estradiol on human breast cancer cells in culture. Cancer Res 1983 (43):349-354
12. De Bortoli ME, Abou-Issa H, Haley BE and Cho-Chung YS: Amplified expression of p21 ras protein in hormone-dependent mammary carcinoma of humans and rodents. Biochem Biophys Res Commun 1985 (127):699-706
13. Dickson RB, Huff KK, Spencer EM and Lippman ME: Introduction of epidermal growth factor-related polypeptides by 17 ß -estradiol in MCF-7 human breast cancer cells. Endocrinology 1986 (118):138-142
14. Dupont WD and Page DL: Risk factors for breast cancer in women with proliferative breast disease. New Engl J Med 1985 (312):146-151
15. Fitzpatrick SL, Brightwell J, Wittliff JL, Barrows GH and Schultz GS: Epidermal growth factor binding by breast tumor biopsies and relationship to estrogen receptor and progestin receptor. Cancer Res 1984 (44):3448-3453
16. Fitzpatrick SL, LaChance MP and Schultz GS: Characterization of epidermal growth factor receptor and action on human breast cancer cells in culture. Cancer Res 1984 (4):3442-3447
17. Foulds L: Neoplastic Development. 1969 (1):46-90 London: Academic Press
18. Glaichenhaus N, Mougneau E, Connan G, Rassoulzadegan M and Cuzin F: Cooperation between multiple oncogenes in rodent embryo fibroblasts: an experimental model of tumor progression. Adv Cancer Res 1985 (45):291-305
19. Goustin AS, Leof EB, Shipley GD and Moses HL: Growth factors and cancer. Cancer Res 1986 (46):1015-1029
20. Green S, Walter P, Kumar V, Krust A, Bornert JM, Argos P and Chambon P: Human oestrogen receptor cDNA: sequence expression and homology to v- erb-A. Nature 1986 (320):134-139
21. Greene GL, Gilna P, Waterfield M, Baker A, Hort Y and Shine J: Sequence and expression of human estrogen receptor complementary DNA. Science 1986 (231):1150-1154
22. Jaspar JM and Franchimont P: Radioimmunoassay of human

epidermal growth factor in human breast cyst fluid. Eur J Cancer Oncol 1985 (21):1343-1348

23. Jensen HM, Chen I, DeVault MR and Lewis AE: Angiogenesis induced by 'normal' human breast tissue: a probable marker for precancer. Science 1982 (218):293-295
24. Haslam SZ: Mammary fibroblast influence on normal mouse mammary epithelial cell responses to estrogen in vitro. Cancer Res 1986 (46):310-316
25. Horwitz KB, Wei LL, Sedlacer SM and d'Arville CN: Progestin action and progesterone receptor structure in human breasr cancer: a review. Recent Prog Horm Res 1985 (41):249-316
26. Kasid A, Lippman ME, Papageorge AG, Lowy DR and Gelman EP: Transfection of v- rasH DNA into MCF-7 human breast cancer cells bypasses dependece on estrogen for tumorigenicity. Science 1985 (228):725-728
27. Kim U and Depowski MJ: Progression from hormone dependence to autonomy in mammary tumors as an in vivo manifestation of sequential clonal selection. Cancer Res 1975 (35):2068-2077
28. King RJB: How important are steroids in regulating the growth of mammary tumors? In: Litwack G (ed): Biochemical action of hormones 1979 (6):247-264 New York: Academic Press
29. King RJB: Effects of female sex hormones on human endometrium in relation to neoplasia. In: Lewis GP and Ginsburg M (eds) Mechanisms of Steroid Action 1981 49-58 London: Macmillan
30. King RJB, Coffer AI, Gilbert J, Lewis K, Nash R, Millis R, Raju S and Taylor RW: Histochemical studies with a monoclonal antibody raised against a partially purified soluble estradiol receptor preparation from human myometrium. Cancer Res 1985 (45):5728-5733
31. King RJB, Kaye AM and Shodell MJ: Copurification of an oestrogen-induced protein from rat uterus and a factor able to stimulate DNA synthesis in cultured cells. Exp Cell Res 1977 (109):1-8
32. King RJB and Mainwaring WIP: Steroid-cell interactions. London Butterworths 1974
33. King RJB and Whitehead MI: Estrogen and progestin effects on epithelium and stroma from pre- and postmenopausal endometria: application to clinical studies of the climacteric syndrome. In: Jasonni VM, Nenci I and Flamigni C (eds): Progress in cancer research and therapy. 1983 : 105-115 New York: Raven Press
34. Klein G and Klein E: Evolution of tumours and the impact of molecular oncology. Nature 1985 (315):190-195
35. Lippman M: Hormonal regulation of human breast cancer cells in vitro. In: Pike MC, Siiteri and Welsch CW (eds): The Banburry Report 1981 : 171-181 Cold Spring Harbor Laboratory
36. Lippman ME, Dickson RB, Kasid A, Gelmann E, Davidson N, McManaway M, Huff K, Bronzert D, Bates S, Swain S and Knabbe C: Autocrine and paracrine growth regulation of human breast cancer. J Steroid Biochem 1986 (24):147-154
37. McGrath M, Palmer S and Nandi S: Differential response of normal rat mammary epithelial cells to mammogenic hormones and EGF. J Cell Physiol 1985 (125):181-191
38. Miesfeld R, Okret S, Wikstrom AC, Wrange O, Gustafsson JA and Yamamoto KE: Characterization of a steroid hormone receptor gene and mRNA in wild-type and mutant cells. Nature 1984 (312):779-781

39. Murphy LJ, Sutherland RL, Stead B, Murphy LC and Lazarus L: Progestin regulation of epidermal growth factor receptor in human mammary carcinoma cells. Cancer Res 1986 (46):728-734
40. Mukku VR and Stancel GM: Regulation of epidermal growth factor receptor by estrogen. J Biol Chem 1985 (260):9820-9824
41. Northrop JP, Gametchu B, Harrison RW and Ringold GM: Characterization of wild type and mutant glucocorticoid receptors from rat hepatoma and mouse lymphoma cells. J Biol Chem 1985 (260):6398-6403
42. O'Neill C, Jordan P and Ireland G: Evidence for two distinct mechanisms of anchorage stimulation in freshly explanted and 3T3 Swiss mouse fibroblast. Cell 1986 (44):489-496
43. Page DL, Dupont WD, Rogers IW and Rados MS: Atypical hyperplastic lesions of the female breast. A long-term follow-up study. Cancer 1985 (55):2698-2708
44. Perel E, Daniilescu D, Kharlip L, Blackstein ME and Killinger DW: The relationship between growth and andro-stenedione metabolism in four cell lines of human breast carcinoma cells in culture. Mol Cell Endocrinol 1985 (41):197-203
45. Reddel RR, Murphy LC, Hall RE and Sutherland RL: Differential sensitivity of human breast cancer cell lines to the growth-inhibitory effects of tamoxifen. Cancer Res 1985 (45):1525-1531
46. Roberts AB and Sporn MB (eds):Cancer Surv (4) 1985
47. Robert AB and Sporn MB: Trasforming growth factors. Cancer Surv 1985 (4):683-706
48. Rochefort H, Capony F, Cavalie-Barthez G, Chanbon M, Garcia M, Massot O, Morisset M, Touitou I, Vignon F and Westley B: Estrogen-regulated protein and autocrine control of cell growth in breast cancer. In: Rich MA, Hager JC and Taylor-papadimitriou J (eds): Breast cancer: origins, detection and treatment. Boston 1986 :57-68 Martinus Nijhoff Publishing
49. Roos W, Fabbro D, Kung W, Costa SD, Eppenberger U: Correlation between hormone dependency and the regulation of epidermal growth factor receptor by tumor promoters in human mammary carcinoma cells. Proc Natl Acad Sci Usa 1986 (83):991-995
50. Rose DP: Endogenous hormones in the etiology and clinical course of breast cancer. In: Rose DP (ed) Endocrinology of cancer 1979 (1):22-52 Boca Ration: CRC press
51. Rozengurt E, Sinnett-Smith J and Taylor-Papadimitriou J: Production of PDGF-like growth factory by breast cancer cell lines. Int J Cancer 1985 (36):247-252
52. Sager R: Genetic suppression of tumor formation. Adv Cancer Res 1985 (44):43-69
53. Sainsbury JRC, Malcolm AJ, Appleton DR, Farndon JR, Harris AL: Presence of epidermal growth factor receptor as an indicator of poor prognosis in patients with breast cancer. J CLin Pathol 1985 (38):1225-1228
54. Sibley CH and Yamamoto KR: Mouse lymphoma cells: mechanisms of resistence to glucocorticoids. In: Baxter JD and Rousseau GG (eds) Monographs on endocrinology 198 (12):357-376
55. Sirbasku DA, Ikeda T and Danielpour D: Endocrine and autocrine estromedins for mammary and pituitary tumor cells. In: Ford RJ and Maizel AL (eds) Mediators in Cell Growth and Differentiation 1985: 213-232 New York: Raven Press

56. Smith HS, Wolman SR, Auer G and HAckett Aj: Cell culture studies: a perspective on malignant progression of human breast cancer. In: Rich MA, Hager JC and Taylor-Papadimitriou J (eds) Breast cancer: origins, detection and treatment 1986 :75-89 Boston: Martinus Nijhoff Publishing
57. Solomon E: Recessive mutation in aetiology of Wilms' tumour. Nature 1984 (309):111-112
58. Sporn MB and Roberts AB: Autocrine paracrine and endocrine mechasisms of growth control. Cancer Surv 1985 (4):627-632
59. Stewart TA, Pattengale PK and Leder P: Spontaneous mammary adenocarcinomas in transgenic mice that carry and express MTV/ myc fusion genes. Cell 1984 (38):627-637
60. Stoker MGP, Pigott D, Taylor-Papadimitriou J: Response to epidermal growth factors of cultured human mammary epithelial cells from benign tumours. Nature 1976 (264):764-767
61. Stoscheck CM and King LE: Role of epidermal growth factor in carcinogenesis. Cancer Res 1986 (46):1030-1037
62. Sukumar S, Notario V, Martin-Zanca D and Barbacid M: Induction of mammary carcinomas in rats by nitroso-methylurea involves malignant activation of H-ras-1 by single point mutations. Nature 1983 (306):658-661
63. Sutherland RL, Murphy LC, Hall RE, Reddel RR, Watts CKW and Taylor IW: Effects of antioestrogens on human breast cancer cells in vitro. Interaction with high affinity intracellular binding sites and effects on cell proliferation kinetics. In: Bresciani F. King RJB, Lippman ME, Namer M and Raynaud JP (eds) Hormone and cancer, progress in cancer research therapy 1983 (31):193-212
64. Thomas DB: Do hormones cause breast cancer? Cancer 1984 (53):595-604
65. Vic P, Vignon F, Derocq and Rochefort H: Effect of estradiol on the ultrastructure of the MCF7 human breast cancer cells in culture. Cancer Res 1982 (42):667-673
66. Viola MV, Fromowitz F, Oravez S, Deb S, Finkel G, Lundy J, Hand P, Thor and Scholm J: Expression of ras oncogene p21 in prostate cancer. New Engl J Med 1986 (314):133-137
67. Weinberg RA: The action of oncogenes in the cytoplasm and nucleus. Science 1985 (230):770-776
68. Weiberg C, Hollenberg SM, Rosenfeld MG and Eveans RM: Domain structure of human glucocorticoid receptor and its relationships to the v-erb-A oncogene product. Nature 1985 (318):670-672
69. Welsch CW: Factors affecting the growth of carcinogen-induced rat mammary carcinomas: a review and tribute to Charles Brenton Huggins. Cancer Res 1985 (45):3415-3443
70. Westphal HM, Mugele K, Beato M and Gehring U.: Immunochemical characterization of wild-type and variant glucocorticoid receptors by monoclonal antibodies.
71. Yates J, Couchman JR and King RJB: Androgen effects on growth morphology and sensitivity of S115 mouse mammary tumor cells in culture. In: Iacobelli S, King RJB, Lindner HR and Lippman ME: Hormone and cancer, progress in cancer research and therapy 1980 (14):31-39 New york: Raven Press
72. Yates J and King RJB: Correlation of growth properties and morphology with hormone responsivwness of mammary tumor cells in culture. Cancer Res 1981 (41):258-262

73. Zachary I and Rozengurt E: Modulation of the epidermal growth factor receptor by mitogenic ligands: effects of bombesin and role of protein kinase C. Cancer Surv 1985 (4):729-766
74. Zwiebel JA, Bano M, Nexo E, Salomon DS and Kidwell WR: Partial purification of transforming growth factors from human milk. Cancer Res 1986 (46):933-939
75. Zwiebel JA, Davis MR, Kohn E, Salomon DS and Kidwell WR: Anchorage-independent growth-conferring factor production by rat mammary tumor cells. Cancer Res 1982 (42):5117-5125

Steroids, Growth Factors and Oncogenes in Breast Cancer

S. Saez

Centre Leon Berard, 28, rue Laennec, Lyon, France

In spite of recent dramatic advances in the knowledge of general carcinogenesis and in spite also of the availability of very active chemotherapeutic agents, all cancers cannot be cured even if they are treated at an early stage. Breast cancer is one of the tumors for which the long-term outcome remains difficult to predict and to monitor. Many medical groups have outlined rational protocols for adjuvant therapy at early stages. With this approach the disease-free period after treatment of the primary tumor has been extended and the quality of life during that time has been improved. Nevertheless there are still patients whose unfavorable outcome seems to be unchanged by the treatment and who die from extended disease.

There is a strong correlation between stage of disease and pronosis. However, this correlation does not imply that all patients included in the same stage, receiving the same treatment, will benefit to the same extent. The real outcome of any individual case may be worse or better than expected. It is likely that parameters related to biological characteristics of the tumor itself and to its host modulate the course of the disease. Such a hypothesis may be drawn from experimental investigations using cell lines from human origin but there is, as yet, no direct application to individual tumors and their treatment.

For a long time, estrogens have been considered to have a positive effect on breast tumor growth. Many experiments and clinical data support this point of view (1). Estrogenic activity was the first to be indentified but it cannot be dissociated from the hypothalamo-hypophysal system regulating ovarian, adrenal and breast functions (gonodotropins, ACTH, prolactin, growth hormone). A number of clinical studies identified so-called hormone dependent and hormone independent tumors, depending on the success or failure of either hormonal suppression (removal of the sources of estrogens or their stimulines) or administration of hormones able to reduce the expression of estrogenic activity (progestins, androgens).

It is probable that estrogens may play a role in breast cancer growth at different levels. At the level of carcinogenesis itself, there is evidence that their role is restricted to that of cocarcinogen or promotor (1). During tumor growth, it is now admitted that their direct stimulating activity is minimal. Local hormones (growth factors) have been identified which are secreted by estrogen target cells and are under the control of the estrogens themselves. It is a new insight into the mechanism of hormone dependency. Such processes also exist in normal cells (2). It is likley that alternatively or in addition to estrogens other hormones may induce such autocrine stimulation of breast cancer growth (3). In malignant cells, there are defects in the regulation of this system, which are responsible for excessive growth. Nevertheless, the dependency on estrogens would be mediated via the estrogen-receptor mechanism of the target cells.

STEROID RECEPTORS IN TUMORS FROM TARGET AND NON TARGET ORGANS

In the late sixties Jensen reported that measurement of estrogen-receptors (ER) in a tumor biopsy specimen was useful in predicting the response to adrenal surgery (4). Further extensive investigations largely confirmed this observation (5). In the following years it became clear that not all tumors containing ER were hormone dependent and that the simultaneous presence of ER and progesterone receptors (PGR) was of greater value in defining hormone dependency. This hypothesis had been previously put forward by Horwitz et al (7) since PGR itself is dependent on estrogens and on the estrogen-receptor machinery for its synthesis in target cells.

In the light of these observations, the hypothesis suggesting the existence of two varieties of tumors seemed logical: 1. those which retain hormone receptors normally present in the mammary gland and which are hormone-dependent. 2. those which lose their receptors possibly as a result of malignant transformations and which are no longer able to respond to the hormonal message. Extensive studies of estrogen and progesterone receptors in primary tumors have been performed by many laboratories and medical groups. They led to another assessment which turned out be in perfect agreement with the very early clinical observations: statistical analyses of the relationship between the patient outcome to the receptor status of the tumor established that recurrence was less frequent in patients whose tumors contained ER, and that the mean duration of the disease free interval was longer. This conclusion provided an objective basis for the clinical observations which had previously related the hormone dependent behaviour of the tumors to a good prognosis.

Later on it was reported that the presence of PGR was more significant of favorable long term prognosis than ER alone.

Analysis of parameters which are classically related to growth rate, such as labeling index (9), mitotic index (9), aspects of cell differentiation, provided evidence that the tumors with positive steroid receptor status express characteristics resembling those of the normal original tissue (7).

As the methodology for steroid receptor measurement was relatively simple, it has been applied to the study of a variety of human tumors. The underlying hypothesis was in many cases based on a rapid assimilation of these tumors to the model of breast cancer where there is a strict correlation between the presence of ER/PGR and the stimulatory effect of the corresponding hormones on tumor growth. However, the data obtained so far have been found to be inconsistent with those on tumors from steroid target cells.

Indeed the majority of the tumors which were investigated were not derived from tissues which could be considered targets for steroid hormones, since neither the specific activity nor their morphology was dependent on the activity of these hormones. In some cases epidemiological observations have suggested that sex hormones might play a role in some types of tumor development: melanoma, colonic epithelioma, renal tumors, lymphoma.

These examples merit more detailed comment.

1. Several observations on the natural history of <u>human malignant melanoma</u> have suggested that sex hormones may influence the behaviour of the tumor, its initial development and its growth (11,12). ER, PGR and androgen receptors have been measured in tumor tissue biopsies (13,14), and found to be detectable in about 20% of the cases. Their biochemical characteristics were found to be similar to those of target organs but in general the ER content was lower than that in breast tumors. The authenticity of these ERs has been the subject of controversy due to the affinity of estrogens for tyrosinase. However, the presence of ER has subsequently been confirmed and it is now admitted that ER and other steroid receptors are occasionally present in melanoma tissue. In spite of these observations there are no clear explanations as to the exact role of estrogens in clinical observations and in <u>in vitro</u> experiments. On the one hand the more favorable prognosis is consistent with estrogens inhibiting the growth of ER+ cell lines (15), on the other, dramatic remissions or no objective remissions at all of the lesions have been observed after anti-estrogen treatment (16,17,18).

These apparently conflicting observations may find a possible explanation in the results of Chaudhury (13), who observed that ERs were detected in benign naevi in normal subjects but were present only in benign naevi from patients with melanoma. This would suggest that ERs could be present as a result of one of the multiple changes occuring during the process of cell transformation, but it does not provide any decisive argument in favor of their activity on growth.

Recent investigations have demonstrated biochemical activities which could be linked to unregulated growth: the production of a TGF α like transforming activity and of a monolayer mitogen (19), the characterization of Nerve Growth Factor receptors (20).

<u>Colonic epithelioma</u> represents an interesting model since data on steroid receptors are available in normal and tumor tissues from human biopsies and animal experiments (21,22,23). Epidemiological observations in human and animal carcinogenesis experiments suggest that sex hormones may play a role in the development of adenocarcinoma in the colonic mucosa, which is not an active target organ for these hormones. Androgen receptors (AR) have been reported in dimethylhydrazine (DMH) induced colonic cancers in rats (22,23). ER and PGR were determined with the same incidence in animals of both sexes. It was observed that ARs

become detectable during and after tumorigenesis, but the effect of castration and androgen administration on tumor incidence in male and female rats is controversial.

In humans, steroid receptors in apparently normal mucosa are found more frequently in biopsies from patients affected with colonic cancer than in those from normal subjects (24). It appears reasonable, therefore, to suggest that androgens might influence the promotion or progression rather than the initiation of carcinogenesis. Their receptors would be expressed only in the transformed tissue. This point of view is consistent with the observation tARs reach their highest level in the established tumor.

Curiously, epidemiological data show that colorectal and renal cancers have a similar distribution as breast cancer in humans (25,26).

<u>Experimental</u> <u>renal</u> tumors may be provoked in the castrated male Chinese Hamster by continuous diethylstilbestrol (DES) administration (27). During the several passages in homologous animals, they become independent of hormone treatment and they acquire steroid receptors at the same time (ER, PGR, AR). The PGR content is very elevated and its level remains sensitive to oestrogen treatment (29,29,30). The effectiveness of hormonal administration in reducing tumor growth rate is related to its capacity to decrease the ER content (31). In spite of the epidemiological data and some confirmative investigations, it is more difficult to relate the clinical course of human disease to sex steroid activities (32,33). No hormonal treatment has been proven to be effective at an acceptable rate.

Non-epithelial tumors also have been induced after estrogen administration: after long-term treatment which elicits a permanent prolactin hypersecretion, <u>lymphomas</u> have been obtained in Nb rats. They are at first dependent on estrogen treatment and later become independent (34). An Nb2 lymphoma cell line has been established from these tumors. It contains receptors specific for prolactin and lactogenic hormones and these hormones effectively stimulate its growth (35,36). It is also sensitive to hCG, an oncofetal hormone which may be the product of ectopic synthesis by a variety of tumors (37).

In those malignant tumors, originally developed by estrogen treatment, this acquired sensitivity to polypeptide hormones and the expression of the corresponding receptors might be the result of malignant transformation.

From these observations, it can be assumed that changes in hormone receptor content may be associated with the transformation process. The hypothesis, indicated above, which suggests that the presence of steroid receptors in tumors from target organs is a reflection of the similarity between the tumor and the normal tissue from which it is derived, should be modulated in view of the data obtained on non-target organ tumors.

In adenocarcinoma from estrogen and progesterone target organs, analysis of the mean content in receptors indicates that PGR is related to the amount of ER. In our experience, we have observed from the analyses of individual cases that the presence of PGR is a better index of hormone dependency than a high level of ER. We have observed that very high contents in ER may be found in breast tumors which do not express PGR and which do not exhibit a differentiated morphology. Similar features were found in endometrium adenocarcinoma. Indeed we found that the presence of PGR is associated with a moderate content of ER and that this pattern corresponds to the differentiated cytological aspect.

Not all breast and endometrium adenocarcinomas contain steroid receptors. Therefore, either a loss or an increase iptor content could be associated with cell transformation (38). PGRs effectively express the persistence of ER specialized activity. We suggest that a differentiated morphology would be the consequence of hormone activity, which itself can be mediated by the receptors and the cell machinery.

In malignant target cells hormone receptors are either absent or, if present, their content may be lower or higher than that in normal tissue. In the first case, tumor cells are not even able to detect the hormonal message. In the second case they can detect it but may or may not express the corresponding activity, depending on the maintenance of related cellular structures. In non-target tissue, the induction of receptors during the process of carcinogenesis would be due to the same mechanism(s), responsible for the synthesis of inappropriate proteins and which has been well documented. It has been recognized that these proteins are "markers" of malignancy. They may be endowed with biological activity depending on the presence of the other parameters necessary for the complete pathway.

This activity may be a specific cellular function or may be involved in the induction of growth. We have previously seen that steroid receptors mediate this double role. On the one hand they participate in relation with other hormones in the specific function of their target cells. On the other hand they stimulate the production of peptides which are active in promoting cell growth. Such cell growth may theoretically be monitored by appropriate hormonal treatment.

GROWTH FACTORS AND ONCOGENE PRODUCTS

The growth factors (GF) produced in the so-called hormone dependent or hormone independent tumors are very similar to those which are responsible for regulating growth. In malignant cells they are able to maintain the growth regulatory mechanism permanently turned on when they act at the wrong time or in the wrong place (40,41,42).

They represent one variety of transforming agents or <u>oncogene products</u> in malignant cells. They constitute an altered version of the normal proteins and they induce impaired activities. During the past few years, several kinds of oncogene products have been identified and related to the key function of the cell growth pathway where they are active.

- they can mimick the activity of the growth factors which regulate differentiation or division. The product is synthesized by the malignant cell and is active through an autocrine mechasism (39).
- they can be growth factor receptors with structural and functional homologies with "transforming" protein kinases which mediate the polypeptide growth activity.
- they may be responsible for changes in normal cell activity at a more distal, post receptor point in the growth pathway.

In normal 3T3 cells (43), the successive activities of several factors which belong to different families are necessary for promoting growth and division which is the result of the progression of the cell into the cycle.
At the earliest stage of the cycle, Platelet Derived Growth Factor (PDGF) and Fibroblast Growth Factor (FGF) induce a state of competence to cells arrested to G0.
The Epidermal Growth Factor (EGF) acts on competent cells and drives them from G0 to G1.
The late progression from G1 up to S is dependent upon somatomedins.

GROWTH FACTORS - ONCOGENE PRODUCTS - STEROID RECEPTORS

Breast tumor cell lines and tumor biopsies of human origin possess receptors for somatomedin-C and EGF (44,45,46), independently of the presence of steroid receptors (45,47) and they respond to addition of these GF in vitro by an increase in growth (44,46,47,48). Furthermore, production of Somatomedin-C and EGF related factor has been observed in one cell line. The factor related to EGF presumably belongs to the
-TGF family and its production is increased by estradiol (49,50). These experiments clearly establish the potential indirect role of steroid molecules on growth and their link with the functioning of polypeptide growth factors.
This indirect role is not restricted to non peptide hormones since prolactin may also stimulate autocrine production of growth factors (10).

These observations are examples of malignant introduction of paranormal GFs in the cell growth process. These factors belong to the same families in both cases but their release may alternatively exhibit dependency or independency on identified hormones.

The activities of these factors being dependent on their receptors, EGF-receptors (EGF-R) have been investigated in a variety of tissues. In breast tumors EGF-R are not always present (45,47,51). They are found independently of the ER/PGR status but their content is more elevated in ER/PGR negative tumors (45/47). In breast tumors (52), like in other tumors, the induction of or increase in EGF-R expression may be related to transformation (53,54,55). EGF-R mediates growth stimulation (48) or inhibition (51,52) of breast tumors in vitro, depending on the variety of cells and on the dose of EGF.

While RGF-R is positively regulated by estradiol in the rat uterus (56), by dexamethasone in Hela S3 cells (57), progestins have been found to be the most effective steroid in provoking a rapid increase in EGF-R and lactogenic receptors (58,59). This effect is observed in human cell lines in which PGR content is d to ER activity. It is quantitatively related to the amount of PGR present in the cell line and to the affinity of the steroid with PGR. In another cell line progestins elicit an increase in insulin receptors and a growth inhibitory activity (60).

In the model of hen oviduct, purified preparation of insulin and RGF are active in phosphorylating the progesterone receptor with high affinity at tyrosine residues. EGFs preferentially phosphorylate the 80-K Da and 105-k Da subunits while insulin preferentially phospohorylates the 80-K Da (61,63). This activity could provide a mechanism for transmitting the EGF signal to the nuclear sites recognized by progesterone receptors. At the same time, phosphorylation of the steroid receptors is an obligatory step for their nuclear activity.

The avian PGR is indistinguishable, by several methods of analysis, from either a 90-K Da protein which complexes with the Rous Sarcoma Virus protein pp v-src, or from the major heat shock protein. This 90-K Da protein complexes also to avian estrogen, androgen and glucocorticoid receptors (63).

These observations represent a link between the activity of steroid and polypeptide hormones, between steroid receptors and viral proteins, but their complete significance is not elucidated.

Recent investigations provide further insight into the relationship between growth factors, oncogenes and steroid receptors.

It has been shown that the v-erb-B gene from Avian Erythroblastosis virus (AEV) codes for the cytoplasmic domain of EGF-R which does not bind EGF and is responsible for the autophosphorylation of the receptor. V-erb-A potentiates the action of V-erb-B by a known mechanism.

The cDNAs of human glucocorticoid and estrogen receptors have been cloned recently (64,65). It is shown that the human glucocorticoid receptor (GR) is related to the v-erb-A oncogene product of AEV. The region with maximal homology with erb-A corresponds to a cysteine-lysine-argin rich portion of the receptor and it is assumed that this zone corresponds to the GR-DNA binding domain.

It was also shomn that there is extensive homology between the ER-cDNA and the erb-A gene of the AEV. The corresponding region is also found to be rich in cystein, lysine and arginine. It is reactive with the H 226 monoclonal ER antibody which recognizes the epitope localized in the DNA-binding domain of the molecule.

The homology of both receptors sequences with erb-A and their localization at an active region which could correspond to the

DNA-binding domain suggest that the oncogenicity of AEV could be explained by the inappropriate activity of an altered steroid receptor molecule, or a related regulatory molecuoded by v-erb-A (60).

The H.ras gene from the Harvey Murine Saroma Virus has an oncogenic potential. A similar gene has been identified in a nitroso-methylurea (NMU) induced breast tumor (66). It belongs to a family of 3 related genes, identified also in human tumors. They code for highly related proteins called pp.^{21}.
These experiments raise the question of the role of chemical carcinogens in oncogene activation in human neoplasia.
Experiments on transfection of v-ras-H DNA into MCF-7 cells have been carried out (67). In contrast to the parental cell line, MCF-7 ras cell no longer responded to exogenous oestrogens in culture and demonstrated a low sensitivity to antiestrogens. Tested in nude mice, MCF-7 ras was fully tumorigenic in the absence of estrogen supplementation. Nevertheless, MCF-7 ras cells still contained ER and estrogen inducible PGR, but their main growth activity was dependent on v-ras infection.

Further experiments have shown that an enhanced expression of c-ras H oncogene, p21 transforming proteins, is associated with hormone dependent growth of DMBA rat mammary tumors while hormone deprivation which elicits tumor regression reduces the expression of p21 proteins (68). The expression of p21 is not elevated in experimental independent tumors, suggesting that p21 might play a role in the growth of hormone-dependent breast cancer. The presence of gp52 related antigen, the product of MuMTV, in human mammary carcinoma indicates an immunological relationship between human and murine carcinoma (68,69,70). MuMTV tumors are known to be related to glucocorticoid activity in mice and in <u>in vitro</u> experiments. There is apparently no relationship between the expression of MuMTV protein in human tumors, the presence of steroid receptors and hormone dependency (69,71). But the infection of heterologous cells with MuMTV leads to an increased capacity for anchorage-independent growth mediated by insulin, and to induction of the expression of p52 protein (70).

Most of these experiments are related to growth factors which are active at the progression state of the cell cycle. They are concerned with EGF-like factors or protein kinase able to activate the cycle.

There are few data on competence factor activity in breast tumors. C-myc expression is not frequent in breast tumors (71) but experiments showing that its micro-injection into quiescent 3T3 cells exposed to platelet-poor-plasma induces DNA synthesis, indicate that under certain circumstances c-myc could be considered to be a competence factor (72). Other identified oncogenes have not yet been extensively investigated in breast tumors.

Some lines of results obtained in other tumor types could nevertheless suggest a new hypothesis for research on breast tumor cell growth: agents which belong to the vitamin family have been shown to be able to modulate oncogene expression while they reduce growth. (73).

The activity of steroids in human breast cancer has been extensively investigated during the last decade. It is ghly recommended to measure the sex steroid receptors in all breast tumor biopsies. The information obtained by this analysis help to select patients for adjuvant or palliative treatment. But ER and PGR are present in not more than 30-40% of the patients.

Thus it is imperative to improve our knowledge of the biology of hormone independent tumors. More recent data indicate that both hormone independent and hormone dependent tumors present alterations in the regulation of the cell cycle. These alterations involve either the hormones normally responsible for the process or some step in the corresponding cell receptor activity. They are related to the transformation and represent an altered function of a normal process.

It is no longer possible to separate hormone independent from hormone dependent tumors except by the criteria of the presence of sex steroid receptors. Their altered growth pathway is relevant to a similar mechanism. In both kinds of tumors, it is promoted by local growth factors, which are also active in normal growth. The physiological action mechanism of hormones on the target organ may be amplified (hormone dependent) or completely destroyed (hormone independent tumors). Inappropriate properties may also be acquired like in any kind of tumor.

Thus it can be assumed that there are common features between tumors which depend on steroids for their growth and those which do not. There are interferences between the activities of steroid and polypeptide hormones. Oncogene products may represent altered versions of normal protein. When they mimick the activity of proteins normally active in the regulated cell cycle, they promote changes which may impair the growth regulation.

Investigations into this field should provide information which is just as useful as steroid receptors have been in the past for the knowledge of breast cancer. And this might lead to new lines of treatment concerning hormone dependent and hormone independent tumors as well.

REFERENCES

1. Leung BS: Role of estrogen in mammary development tumorigenesis and promotion of tumor growth. In: Leung BS (ed) Hormonal regulation of mammary tumors: steroid hormones 1982 (1):30-72 Eden Press Inc
2. Leland FE, Lio M, Sirbasku D: Hormone-dependent cell lines. In: Functionally differentiated cell lines. 1981: 1-46 New York: Alan Liss ed
3. Manni A, Pontari M, Wright C: Autocrine stimulation by prolactin of hormone-responsive breast cancer growth in culture. Endocrinology 1985 (117):2040-2043
4. Jensen EV, DeSomb Jungblut PW: Estrogen receptors in hormone-responsive tissues and tumours. In: Wissler RW, Dao TL, Wood Jr S (eds) Endogeneous factors influencing host-tumor balance 1968: 15-30 Chicago: University of Chicago Press

5. McGuire WL: Estrogen receptors in human breast cancer. J Clin Invest 1973 (52):73-77
6. Clark G, McGuire WL, Hubay CA, Pearson OH, Marshall JS: Progesterone receptors as a prognostic factor in stage II breast cancer. New Engl J Medicine 1983 (309):1342-1347
7. Horwitz KB, McGuire WL, Pearson OH, Segaloff A: Predicting response to endocrine therapy in human breast cancer. Science 1975 (189):726-727
8. Silvestrini R, Daidone MG, Gasparini G: Cell kinetics as a prognostic marker in node-negative breast cancer. Cancer 1985 (56):1982-1987
9. Meyer JS, McDivitt RW, Stone KR, Prey MU, Bauer WC: Practical breast carcinoma cell kinetics: review and update. Breast Cancer Res Treat 1984 : 79-88
10. Manni A: Hormone receptors and breast cancer. New Engl J Medicine 1983 (309):1383-1385
11. Shaw HM, Milton GW, Farago G, McCarthy WH: Endocrine influence on survival from malignant melanoma. Cancer 1978 (42):669-677
12. Shiu MH, Schottenfeld D, MacLean B, Fortner JG: Adverse effect of pregnancy on melanoma. Cancer 1976 (37):181-187
13. Chaudhuri Pk, Walker MJ, Briele HA, Beattle CW, Das Gupta TK: Incidence of estrogen receptor in benign nevi and human malignant melanoma. JAMA 1980 (244):791-793
14. Neifeld JP, Lippman ME: Steroid hormone receptors and melanoma. J Invest Dermatology 1980 (74):379-381
15. Beattle CW, Chaudhuri Pk, Walker MJ, Das Gupta JK: Hormonal regulation of the growth and metastasis of human melanoma. Cancer Treat Report 1979 (63):1199
16. Mirimanoff RO, Wagenknecht L, Hunziker N: Long-term complete remission of malignant melanoma with tamoxifen. Lancet 1981 (2):1368-1369
17. Gill PG, De Young NJ, Thompson A, Keightley DD, Horsfall DJ: The effect of tamoxifen on the growth of human malignant melanoma in vitro. Europ J Cancer Clin Oncol 1984 (20):807-815
18. Rose C, Pedersen L, Mouridsen HT: Endocrine treatment with anti-estrogen, anti-androgen or progestogen of advanced malignant melanoma: three consecutive phase II trials. Europ J Cancer Oncol 1985 (21):1171-1174
19. Richmond A, Lawson DH, Nixon DW, Chawla RK: Characterization of autostimulatory and transforming growth factors from human melanoma cells. Cancer Research 1985 (45):6390-6394
20. Grob PM, Ross AH, Koprowski H, Bothwell M: Characterization of the human melanoma Nerve Growth Factor receptor. J Biol Chem 1985 (26):8044-8049
21. Alford TC, DO H, Geelhoed GW, Tsa NT, Lippman ME: Steroid hormone receptors in human colon cancers. Cancer 1979 (43):980-984
22. Mehta RG, Fricks CM, Moon RC: Androgen receptors in chemically-induced colon carcinogenesis. Cancer 1980 (45):1085-1089
23. O Dagiri E, Jibiki K, Kato Y, Nakamura S, Oda SI, Demura R, Demura H: Steroid receptors in dimethylhydrazine induced colon carcinogenesis. Cancer 1985 (56):2627-2634
24. Marugo M, Molinari F, Fazzuoli L, Parodi MC, Bernasconi D, Menozzi F and Giordano G: Estradiol and progesterone receptors and pathologic colonic mucosa in human. J Endocrinol Invest 1985 (8):117-119

25. Mac Mahon B, Cole P, Brown J: Etiologie of human breast cancer. J Natl Cancer Inst 1973 (50):21-42
26. Howell MA: The association between colorectal cancer and breast cancer. J Chronic Dis 1976 (29):243-261
27. Kirkman H: Autonomous derivates of estrogen-induced renal carcinomas and spontaneous renal tumors in the Syrian hamster. Cancer Research 1974 (34):2728-2744
28. Li JJ, Talley DJ, LI SA, Villee CA: Receptor characteristics of specific estrogen binding in the renal adenocarcinoma of the golden hamster. Cancer Research 1976 (36):1127-1132
29. Li J, Cuthbertson TL, LI SA: Specific androgen binding in the kidney and estrogen dependent renal carcinoma of the Syrian hamster. Endocrinology 1977 (101):1006-1015
30. Li J, LI SA, Cuthbertson TL: Nuclear retention of all steroid hormone receptor classes in the hamster renal carcinoma. Cancer Research 1979 (39):2647-2651
31. Li SA, Li JJ: Estrogen-induced progesterone receptor in the Syrian hamster kidney. Modulation by anti-oestrogen and androgens. Endocrinology 1978 (103):2119-2128
32. Mukamel E, Bruais S, Nissenkorn I Servadio C: Steroid receptors in renal cell carcinoma: relevance to hormonal therapy. J Urology 1984 (131):227-230
33. Harris DT: Hormonal therapy and chemotherapy of renal cell carcinoma. Seminars in Oncology 1983 (10):322-430
34. Noble RL, Hochachka BC, King D: Spontaneous and estrogen produced tumors in Nb rats and their behaviour after transplantation. Cancer Research 1975 (35):766-780
35. Gout PW, Beer CT, Noble RL: Prolactin-stimulated growth of cell cultures established from malignant Nb rat lymphoma. Cancer Research 1980 (40):2433-2436
36. Shiu RPC, Esholtz HP, Tanaka T, Friesen HG , Gout PW, Beer CT, Noble RL: Receptor-mediated mitogenic action of prolactin in a rat lymphoma cell line. Endocrinology 1983 (113):159-165
37. Melmed S, Braustein GD: Human chorionic gonadotropin stimulates proliferation of Nb2 rat lymphoma cells. J Clin Endocrinol Metab 1983 (56):1069-1070
38. Cikes M: Expression of hormone receptors in cancer cells: a hypothesis. Europ J Cancer 1978 (14): 211-215
39. Sporn MB, Todaro GJ: Autocrine secretion and malignant transformation on cells. N Engl J Med 1980 (303):878-880
40. The transforming growth factors. Trends in Biochem Sciences 1985 (5067):237-240
41. Heldin CH, Wstermark B: Growth factors: Mechanism of action and relation to oncogenes. Cell 1984 (37):9-20
42. Salomon DS, Zweibel JA, Mozzena S: Presence of transforming growth factors in human breast cancer cells. Cancer Research 1984 (44):4059-4077
43. O'Keefe EJ, Pledger WJ: A model of cell cycle control: sequential events regulated by growth factors. Mol Cell Endocrinol 1983 (31):167-186
44. Furlanetto RW, Di Carlo JN: Somatomedin-C receptors and growth effects in human breast cells maintained in long term culture. Cancer Research 1984 (44):2122-2128
45. Fitzpatrick SL, Brightwell J, Wittliff JL, Barrows GH, Schultz GS: Epidermal Growth Factor binding by breast tumor biopsies and relationship to estrogen receptor and progestin receptor levels. Cancer Research 1984 (44): 3448-3453

46. Fitzpatrick SL, La Chance MP, Schultz GS: Characterization of Epidermal Growth Factor receptor and action on human breast cancer cells in culture. Cancer Research 1984 (44):3442-3447
47. Perez R, Pascual M., Macias A, Lage A: Epidermal growth factor receptors in human breast cancer. Breast Cancer Res Treat 1984 (4):183-193
48. Osborne CK, Hamilton B, Titus G, Livingstone RB: Epidermal growth factor stimulation of human breast cancer cells in culture. Cancer Research 1980 (40):2361-2366
49. Lippman ME: Growth regulation of human breast cancer. Clinical Research 1985 (33):375-382
50. Dickson RB, Huff KK, Lippman ME: Induction of Epidermal growth Factor related polypeptides by 17 ß estradiol in MCF-7 human breast cancer cells. Endocrinology 1986 (118):138-142
51. Imai Y, Leung L, Friesen HG, Shiu RPC: Epidermal Growth Factor receptors and effect of Epidermal Growth Factor on growth of human breast cancer cells in long-term tissue culture. Cancer Research 1982 (42): 4394-4398
52. Filmus J, Pollak MN, Cailleau R, Buick RN: MDA-468, a human breast cancer cell line with a high number of Epidermal Growth Factor (EGF) receptors, has an amplified EGF receptor gene and is growth inhibited by EGF. Biochem Biophys Res Comm 1985 (128):898-906
53. Liberman TA, Razon N, Bartal AD, Schlessinger J, Soreq H: Expression of Epidermal Growth Factor receptor in human brain tumors. Cancer Research 1984 (44):753-760
Reeve SB: Evidence for increased Epidermal Growth Factor receptors in human sarcomas. Int J Cancer 1985 (36):689-693
55. Ozanne B, Schum A, Richard CS, Cassells D, Grossman D, Trent J, Gusterson B, Hendler F: Evidence for increased EGF receptor in epidermal malignancies in cancer cells. Growth factors and transformation Vol III 1985:41-49 Cold Spring Harbor Laboratory New York
56. Mukku VR, Stancel OM: Regulation of Epidermal Growth Factor receptor by estrogen. J Biol Chem 1985 (17):9820-9824
57. Fanger BO, Viceps-Mdore D, Cidlowski JA: Regulation of high and low-affinity Epidermal Growth Factor receptors by glucocorticoids. Archives of Biochem Biophys 1984 (15):141-149
58. Murphy LJ, Sutherland RL, Lazarus L: Regulation of gowth hormone and Epidermal Growth Factor receptor by progestins in breast cancer cells. Biochem Biophys Res Comm 1985 (131):767-773
59. Murphy LJ, Murphy LC, Stead B, Sutherland RL, Lazarus L: Modulation of lactogenic receptors by progetins in cultured human breast cancer cells. J Clin End Metab 1986 (62):280-287
60. Horwitz KB, Freidenberg GR: Growth inhibition and increase of insulin receptors in antiestrogen resistant T-47 D∞ human breast cancer cells by progestin: implication for endocrine therapies. Cancer Research 1985 (45):167-173
61. Ghosh-Dastidar P, Coty WA, Grist RE, Wood DL, Fox GF: Progesterone receptor submits are high affinity substrates for phosphorylation by epidermal growth factor. Proceed Natl Acad Sci 1983 (81):1654-1658
62. Woo DDL, Fay SP, Griest R, Coty W, Goldfine I, Fox CF: Differential phosphorylation of the progesterone receptor by insulin, Epidermal Growth Factor, and Platelet Derived

Growth Factor. J Biol Chem 1986 (261):460-467
63. Schuh S, Yonemoto W, Brugge J, Bauer VJ, Riehl RM, Sullivan WP, Toft DO: A 90.000 dalton binding protein common to both steroid receptors and the Rous Sarcoma virus transforming protein pp 60 v.src. J Biol Chem 1985 (260):14292-14296
64. Weinberger C, Hollenberg SM, Rosenfed MG, Evans RM: Domain structure of human glucocorticoid receptor and its relationships to the v.erb A oncogene product. Nature 1985 (318):670-672
65. Green S, Walter P, Kumar V, Krust A, Bornert JM, Argos P, Chambon P: Human oestrogen receptor cDNA: sequence expression and homology to v.erb.A. Nature 1986 (320):134-139
66. Sukumar A, Notario V, Martin-Zanca D, Barbacid M: Induction of mammary carcinomas in rats by nitroso-methylurea involves activation of H-ras-1 locus by single point mutations. Nature 1983 (306):658-661
67. Kasid A, Lippman ME, Papageorge AG, Lowy DR, Gelmann EP: Transfection of v.ras.H DNA into MCF-7 human breast cancer cells bypasses dependence on estrogen for tumorigenicity. Science 1985 (228):725-728
68. Huang FL, Cho-Chung YS: Hormone-regulated expression of cellular ras^{H} oncogne in mammary carcinomas in rats. Biochem Biophys Res Comm 1984 (123):141-147
69. Levine PH, Mesa-Tejada R, Keydar I, Tabbane F, Spiegelman S, Mourali N: Increased incidence of mouse mammary tumor virus-related antigen in Tunisian patients with breast cancer. Int J cancer 1984 (33):305-308
70. Kryukova IN, Litvinon SV: Hormone-dependent enchancement of neoplastic phenotype expression by MuMTV-infected heterologous cells and MuMTV-induced cellular antigens. Int J Cancer 1984 (33):533-540
71. Kozbor D, Croce CM: Amplification of c.myc oncogene in one of five human breast carcinoma cell lines. Cancer Research 1984 (44):438-441
72. Kasmarek L, Hyland JK, Watt R, Rosenber GM, Baserga R: Micro injected c.myc as a competence factor. Science 1985 (28):1312-1315
73. Amatruda TT, Sidell N, Ranyard J, Koeffler HP: Retinoic acid treatment of human neuroblastoma cells is associated with decreased N.myc expression. Biochem and Biophys Res Comm 1985 (126):1189-1195

Oestrogen and Anti-Oestrogen Action: A Hypothesis for the Regulation of Breast Cancer Cell Replication

V.C. Jordan

Departments of Human Oncology and Pharmacology, Wisconsin Clinical Cancer Center, 600 Highland Avenue, Madison, WI 53792, USA

The aim of this chapter is to affect a synthesis of apparently unrelated observations in different experimental systems, in order to construct a general model of oestrogen action in breast cancer cells. In so doing, potential mechanisms of action of antioestrogens can be formulated, additional therapeutic targets can be identified and reasons for the resistance to antioestrogen therapy can be identified which results in an eventual development of hormone independence. It is clear that one current goal of breast cancer therapy should be to maintain cells in a hormone-dependent state so that their replication can be controlled by specific, relatively non-toxic, antihormonal agents. Rapid hormone-independent growth requires the application of desperate measures to secure additional time for the patient. Chemotherapy, additional surgery and radiotherapy all have significant major side effects which contribute to declining patient morbidity.

Oestrogen produces changes in the biochemistry of the cells in specific tissues (target tissues). Some target cells prefer to replicate (e.g., epithelial cells of the vagina, uterus or certain breast tumours) whereas others predominately respond by increased synthesis of oestrogen-specific products (e.g., lactotrophs in the pituitary gland synthesize and secrete prolactin). As a third alternative, epithelial cells of the uterus and some breast tumours replicate and produce an oestrogen-specific product, the progesterone receptor, which sensitizes the cells to the differentiating effects of progesterone.

Oestrogen produces its effects through an interaction with the oestrogen receptor protein. Oestrogen target tissue may therefore be identified by the demonstration of oestrogen receptor. Normal oestrogen target tissues are composed entirely of those cells which are required to perform a specific task in response to oestrogen stimulation. In contrast, human breast tumours are more often than not heterogeneous mixtures of malignant cells, some of which are not oestrogen responsive. This state of affairs is exemplified by the clinical observation that less than 10% of oestrogen and progesterone receptor negative tumours will respond to endocrine therapy, whereas oestrogen and progesterone receptor positive tumours have an almost 80% probabilty of responding to endocrine therapy. However, a significant number of oestrogen receptor positive tumours are progesterone receptor negative and there is a reduced (30-40%) probability of obtaining an objective response with endocrine therapy. A reason for the clinical observation will be offered as the model for oestrogen action in the hormone-responsive breast cancer cell is developed.

In the model's simplest form (Figure 1) the oestrogen receptors (R_e) are located at multiple gene sites in the nucleus of the cell. For the sake of discussion, one cluster of nuclear oestrogen receptors will be considered to be located at an α site. These oestrogen receptors will control different genes and ultimately different functions than those located at the ß sites. Breast cancer cells, in the absence of exogenous oestrogen, will maintain a fully expanded population of oestrogen receptors and will not express the progesterone receptor which is an oestrogen-regulated protein. Iodinated epidermal growth factor has been found to bind to breast cancer cells; therefore growth factor receptors (GFR) are included on the cell membrane. In fact, it is particularly interesting to note that there is a negative correlation between the number of GFRs observed both in cultured cells and in primary breast tumours (2,3,10) and the presence of oestrogen receptors. Thus oestrogen receptor negative cells have high concentrations of GFRs on their cell surface. This observation raises the question of the relationship of growth factors and steroid hormone receptors (i.e. oestrogen and progesterone receptors).

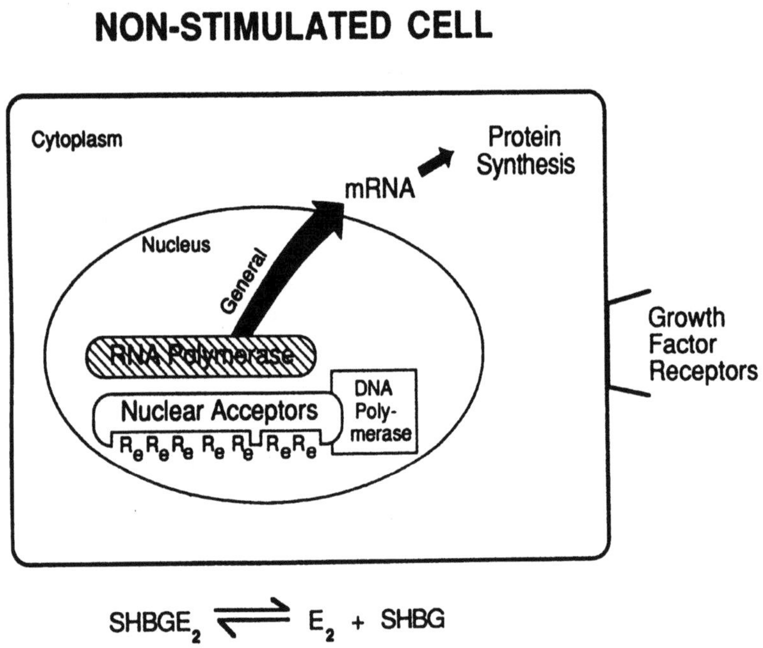

Figure 1. A hypothetical model of oestrogen (E_2) action in the non-stimulated cell. The full oestrogen receptor complement is located in the nucleus for convenience. The α sites (the cluster of receptors on the right of the nuclear acceptor sites) will ultimately control growth factor synthesis. The ß sites are a labile pool of receptors (the cluster on the left of the nuclear acceptors) which will ultimately control additional protein synthetic events to prime the cells for progesterone action. In the non-stimulated cell, growth factors will not occupy the growth factor receptor.

GROWTH FACTOR STIMULATION

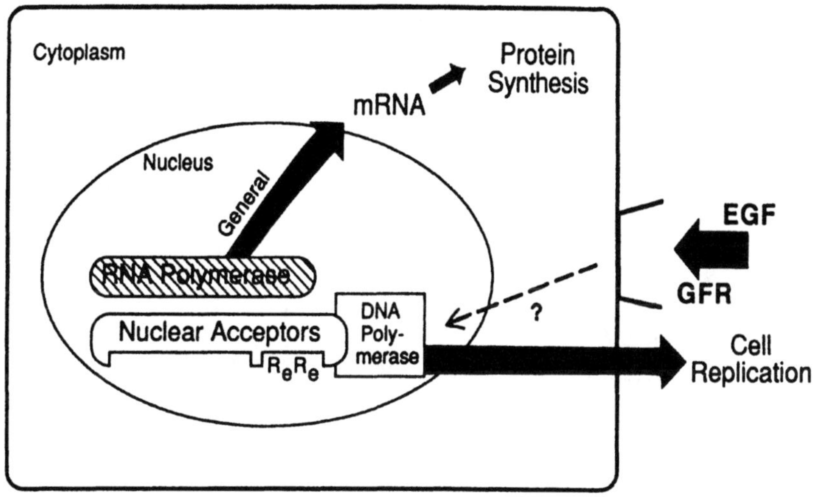

Figure 2. The direct effect of growth factors cause cell replication but also the loss of the ß oestrogen receptor sites. The α sites which would normally control growth factor synthesis are conserved.

Human and mouse epidermal growth factor and rat transforming growth factor alpha all cause a 60% decrease in the level of oestrogen receptors in breast cancer cells in culture (11) (Figure 2). This effect occurs very rapidly and is complete within 6 hourssociated with the decrease in oestrogen receptors is a reduced ability of EGF-treated cells to induce progesterone receptor in response to oestrogen stimulation.

These events could be interpreted as those breast cancer cells that are stimulated to replicate by the growth factor, now choose to reduce the -oestrogen receptor populatiofi at the ß gene site. These sites may, therefore, be involved in non-replication functions and the reduced sensitivity of the cells to progesterone receptor induction by oestrogen supports this view.

Only small concentrations of oestrogen (10^{-12}-10^{-11}-M) are required to increase breast cancer cell replication, whereas larger concentrations of oestrogen (10^{-10}-10^{-9}M) induce progesterone receptor. This implies that there is a differential sensitivity for the nuclear oestrogen receptor sites to activate different sets of genes. Those associated with growth factor synthesis (α sites) are possibly more sensitive to activation than those (ß sites) involved in preparing the cell to differentiate. Thus, given the choice, in a nutrient-rich environment, a breast cancer would prefer to replicate when stimulated by oestrogen.

The possible sequence of events is shown in Figure 3. Oestradiol, which has dissociated from sex hormone binding globulin (SHBG), activates the oestrogen receptors to induce growth factors. The

ESTROGEN STIMULATED GROWTH

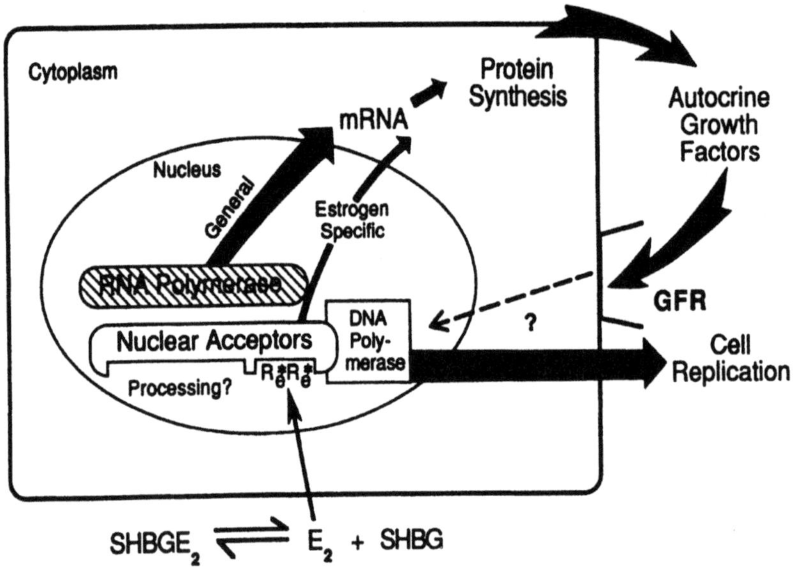

Figure 3. Oestradiol (E_2) dissociates from sex hormone binding globulin (SHBG) to cause cell replication. The effect occurs first in a nutrient-rich environment. The autocrine growth factors cause a decrease in the ß sites (processing).

growth factors initiate events necessary to induce growth factor. The growth factors initiate events necessary to prepare for cell replication, but also decrease oestrogen receptor concentrations. This effects may be the same as "processing" (5,6) that occurs in cultured breast cancer cells within 6 hours of oestrogen stimulation. The cells therefore continue to replicate, unrestricted, as long as the environment remains permissive. Should the levels of growth factors decrease and the cells fail to replicate, then the levels of oestrogen receptors (ß sites) will increase and become available for interaction with oestradiol. Under these conditions of stimulation, progesterone receptor (PgR) would be produced to facilitate the differentiation of the non-replicating cells (Figure 4).

An analogous sequence of events may occur in the uterine cells when increasing oestrogen concentrations cause cell proliferation during the follicular phase of the menstural cycle. However, high concentrations of oestrogen at mid-cycle will prime the cells for the effects of progesterone during the luteal phase.

In a heterogeneous breast tumour, all these different events may be in equilibrium during hormone stimulation. Clones of oestrogen receptor negative tumour cells may produce excessive quantities of growth factors and reduce the oestrogen receptor levels (and ultimately their ability to produce progesterone receptor) in surrounding hormone-dependent cells. Thus oestrogen receptor positive, progesterone receptor negative tumours would occur, but because of the influence of the hormone-independent breast cancer cells, endocrine therapy would, in the majority of cases, be ineffective. Predictably, the best category would be oestrogen and progesterone receptor positive tumours. The mix of tumour cells would be relatively pure, and by expressing the progesterone receptor, they would be demonstrating their slow replicate rate and willingness to differentiate.

The antioestrogen tamoxifen, which is used successfully in breast cancer therapy (4), could interrupt this sequence of events in several ways (Figure 5). Tamoxifen has weak oestrogen-like effects and increases the circulating levels of SHBG. As a result, the concentration of free oestradiol available to diffuse into cells is decreased.

Tamoxifen exhibits a high affinity (Kd 10^{-9} M) interaction with subcellular components referred to as antioestrogen binding sites (AEBS) (14). However, many classes of drugs will bind to AEBS (8), and this interaction may contribute to extend the biological half-life. This is probably a major factor in the seven days biological half-life of tamoxifen.
Tamoxifen inhibits progression of the cell cycle and there is a blockade at the G_1/S interface. Since tamoxifen (and its metabolites) bind to the oestrogen receptor and prevent oestrogen binding in a competitive fashion, high concentrations of the drug are required continually to be present in the target tissue. The drug receptor complex is potentially unable to initiate the synthesis of growth factors required for cell replication. As a result, the level of oestrogen receptors (sites) will increase and some of these will become activated to induce progesterone

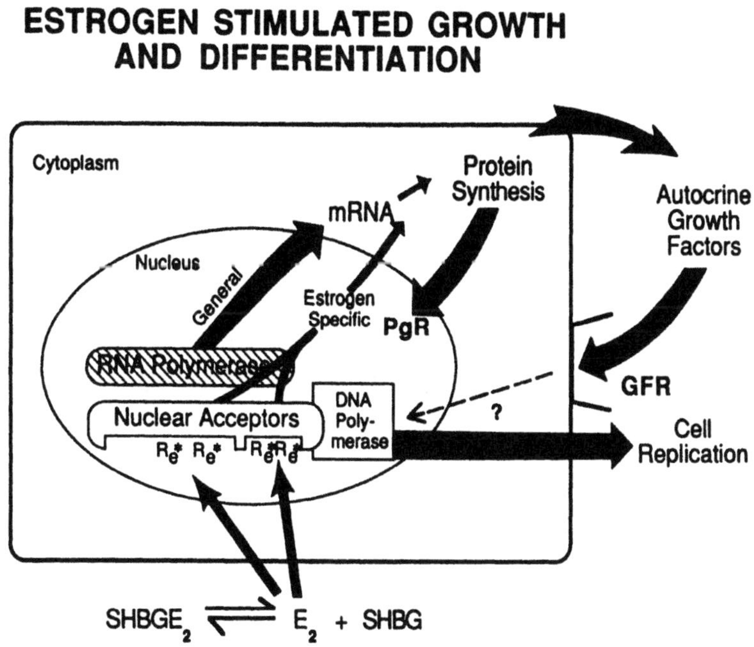

Figure 4. At the equilibrium between resting and proliferating cells, a balance of growth (through α sites) and protein synthesis for differentiation (ß sites) will be established. Progesterone receptor (PgR) will be produced in those cells that do not suffer from the excessive effects of growth factors.

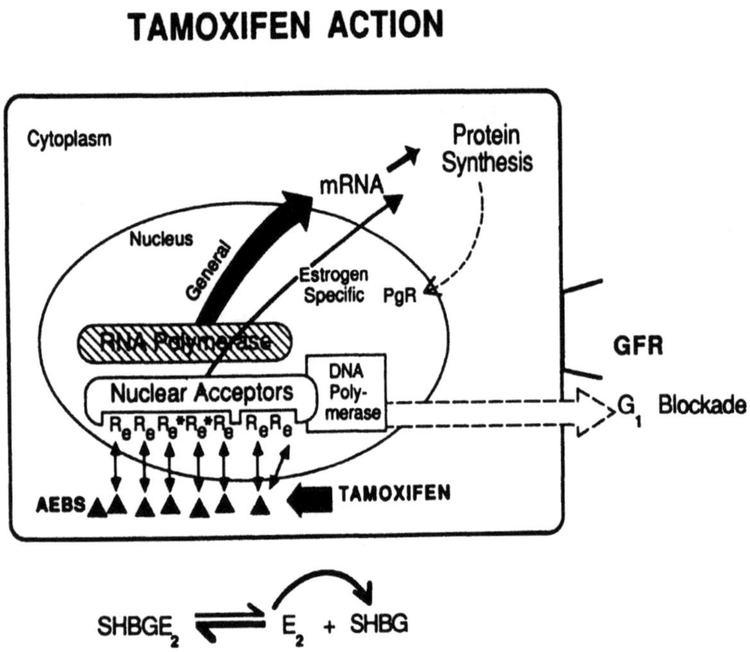

Figure 5. Tamoxifen causes an increase in SHBG; therefore, less E_2 is available to diffuse into the cells. Antioestrogen binding sites (AEBS) will sequester large quantities of tamoxifen and its metabolites and set up an equilibrium to occupy both α and ß oestrogen receptors. Since tamoxifen does not cause the production of growth factors, the result is an increase in oestrogen receptor concentrations and a reversible G_1 blockade of the cell cycle. The ß sites can become partially activated to stimulate some PgR synthesis.

receptors. Therefore, each of the events in the cell are linked by an intimate relationship between both hormone receptor and growth factor systems.

Clearly, tamoxifen will remain an effective agent as long as adequate quantities of the drug remain at a saturating equilibirum on the oestrogen receptor. Tamoxifen therapy will remain effective in homogeneous hormone-responsive tumours for prolonged periods of administration. It is appropriate, therefore, now to consider the failure of the drug based upon the previous proposals and other clinical observations.

Obviously, a competitive antagonist of oestrogen action will fail if oestrogen levels become elevated or the drug levels become too low. The bioavailability of tamoxifen to patients in a low oestrogen environment will become important during prolonged administration (15).

The goal of prolonged therapy must be to prevent the development of hormone-independent clones which will occur if the cells are permitted to replicate. Tamoxifen, however, may become ineffective if growth factors from adjacent cells (normal or malignant) initiate cell division. Drug resistance will, therefore, develop by circumventing the hormone-receptor pathway.

Another possibility is that breast cancer cells adapt to the proliferative effects of another hormone before frank hormone-independence is expressed. One candidate hormone is progesterone. This steroid is generally considered to produce antiproliferative effects in uterine tissues, but there is really no convincing evidence that progestational agents have direct antiproliferative effects on breast cancer cells. In fact, high-dose progestational therapy of breast cancer may act indirectly in vivo by a suppression of adrenal steroidogenesis. It is possible that low doses or physiological doses of progesterone may facilitate tumour development and growth. Early studies with carcinogen-induced rat mammary tumour models demonstrated a positive role for low-dose progesterone administration (1,7) and recently, progestational agents have been shown to increase the concentration of growth factor and prolactin receptors on breast cancer in culture (9). However, to integrate these observations into a model of drug resistance to tamoxifen requires the induction of progesterone receptors in the tissue for progesterone (probably of adrenal origin) to alter the cells and prime them before replication. It is well known that tamoxifen increases progesterone receptor levels; therefore a potential mechanism for progesterone action is available. As yet there are no data concerning the direct actions of progestational agents to facilitate replication in human breast cancer; however, progesterone does reverse the suppressive effects of tamoxifen in the dimethylbenz(a)anthracene-induced rat mammary carcinoma model (12).

Finally, the permissive effects of progesterone to sensitize tamoxifen-treated beast cancer cells to paracine growth factors may provide a working hypothesis to explain the curious efficacy (approximately 50%) of aminoglutethimide in advanced breast cancer patients who have ultimately failed tamoxifen therapy (13). Most research has focused upon the ability of aminoglutethimide to reduce peripheral aromatization of androstenedione to estrogen, and little attention has been paid to the impact on adrenal steroidogenesis. The combined effect of aminoglutethimide and hydrocortisone reduces the availability of pregnenolone to be converted to progesterone (Figure 6). The significance of this effect on the ultimate conversion of breast cancer cells held with tamoxifen to hormone independency should be studied. It is possible from the foregoing discussion that adrenal progesterone, working via the tamoxifen-induced progesterone receptor in the tumour, sensitizes the cells to paracrine growth factors by increasing growth factor receptor levels (9). A decrease in adrenal steroidogenesis would obviously interrupt this sequence of events and produce additional benefit to the patient.

This chapter is offered as a working hypothesis to explain some of the unusual effects observed both in the laboratory and in clinical practice. The balance of cells secreting growth factors in a tumour will determine the hormone receptor status of the tumour and ultimately its ability to respond to antioestrogenic procedures. Furthermore, excessive growth factor secretion will reverse successful antioestrogen therapy. Future strategies to prevent or at least blunt the action of growth factors will provide an additional benefit to control tumour replication.

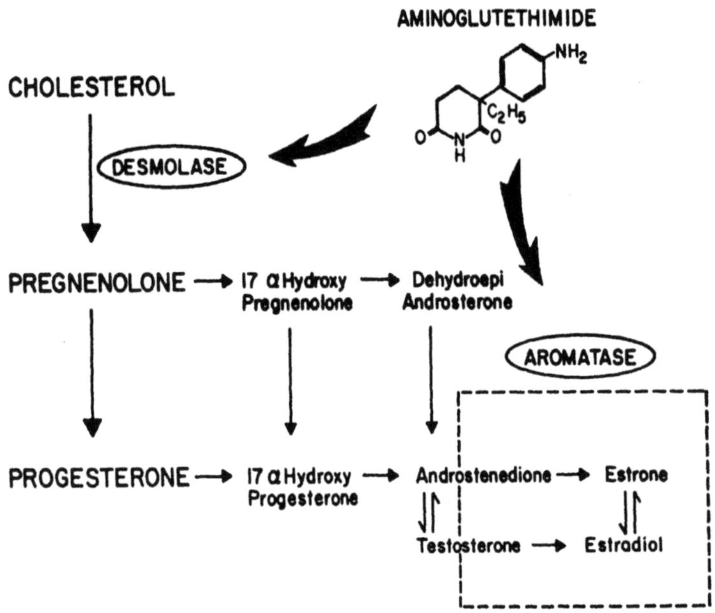

Figure 6. The mode of action of aminoglutethimide on adrenal and peripheral steroidogenesis.

REFERENCES

1. Cantarow A, Stasney J and Paschis KE: The influence of sex hormones on mammary tumors induced by 2-acetaminofluorene. Cancer Res 1984 (8):412-417
2. Fitzpatrick SL, Brightwell J, Wittliff JL, Barrow GH and Schultz GS: Epidermal growth factor binding by breast tumor biopsies and relationship to estrogen and progestin receptor levels. Cancer Res 1984 (44):3448-3453
3. Fitzpatrick SL, Lachance MP and Schultz GS: Characterization of epidermal growth factor receptor and action on human breast cells in culture. Cancer Res 1984 (44):3342-3447
4. Furr BJA and Jordan VC: Pharmacology and clinical uses of tamoxifen. Pharm Therap 1984 (25):127-205
5. Horwitz KB and McGuire WL: Estrogen control of progesterone receptor in human breast cancer. J Biol Chem 1978 (253):2223-2228
6. Horwitz KB, Koseki Y and McGuire WL: Estrogen of progesterone receptor in human breast cancer: role of estradiol and antiestrogen. Endocrinology 1978 (103):1742-1751
7. Huggins C and Young NC: Induction and extinction of mammary cancer. Science 1962 (137):257-262
8. Lyman SD and Jordan VC: Possible mechanisms for the agonist actions of tamoxifen and the antagonist actions of MER-2 (ethamoxytriphetol) in the mouse uterus. Biochem Pharm 1985 (34):2795-2806
9. Murphy LJ, Sutherland, Stead B, Myrphy LC and Lazarus L: Progestin regulations of epidermal growth factor receptor in human mammary carcinoma cells. Cancer Res 1986 (460):728-734
10. Osborne CK, Hamilton B, Titus G and Livingston RB: Receptor binding and processing of epidermal growth factor by human

breast cancer cells. J Clin Endocr Metab 1982 (55):86-93

11. Ravdin PM, Welshons WV and Jordan VC: Regulation of estrogen receptor (ER) levels in human breast cancer cell lines by epidermal growth factor (EGF). Breast Cancer Res Treat 6: Abstract 1985 (57)
12. Robinson SP and Jordan VC: Opposing actions of progesterone and tamoxifen in rats with dimethylbenzathracene (DMBA)-induced rat mammary tumors. Proceedings of the Endocrine Society Anaheim CA 1986.
13. Stuart-Harris RC and Smith IE: Aminoglutethimide in the treatment of advanced breast cancer. Cancer Treat Rev 1984 (11):184-204
14. Sutherland RL, Murphy LC, Foo MS, Green MD, Whybourne AM and Krozowski ZS: High affinity antioestrogen binding site distinct from the oestrogen receptor. Nature (London) 1980 (288):273-275
15. Tormey DC and Jordan VC: Long-term adjuvant therapy in node positive breast cancer - a metabolic and pilot clinical study. Breast Cancer Res Treat 1984 (4):297-302

Methodology of Clinical Trials. Investigating Endocrine Mechanisms in Breast Cancer

R.D. Gelber* and A. Goldhirsch**

*Harvard School of Public Health and Dana-Farber Cancer Institute, Boston, MA, USA
**Ludwig Institute for Cancer Research (Bern Branch), Inselspital, Bern, Switzerland

Clinical trials are widely used to gain information about therapies for patients with cancer. However, adoption of the prospective clinical trial is a fairly recent development. Mike' (1) and Pocock (2) summarize the same historical perspectives in the development of medical investigations.

We define a clinical trial as a scientific experiment conducted with human subjects in which treatments are initiated for the purpose of evaluating one or more therapies. The dictionary defines methodology as the science of method, a way of doing something in an orderly or systematic mode, as in accordance with a definite plan. Methodology of clinical trials then refers to the variety of principles, procedures and techniques that are available to place clinical investigation within an orderly, systematic, and thereby interpretable framework. The clinical trial methodology is designed to provide scientific evidence that is as objective as possible given the inherently subjective aspects of patient care and definition of therapeutic benefit. Several texts that describe aspects of methodologies for clinical trials have appeared recently (2,3,4,5,6).

In the last 20 years, attempts to apply a clinical trial methodology to investigations in the field of breast cancer have provided a variety of noteworthy results (7,8;9). The methodologies applied to <u>study design</u> following the formulation of a clinically relevant question, trial <u>conduct</u>, data <u>analysis</u> and <u>reporting</u> of results influence substantially the reliability and utility of the information obtained. The appropriate interpretation of the findings of any clinical trial must take into consideration how completely and correctly the scientific principles have been applied at each of these four areas.

In this chapter we discuss some general aspects of clinical trial methodology with special emphasis on examples investigating endocrine mechanisms in breast cancer.

OBJECTIVE OF CLINICAL TRIALS

The general objective of the clinical trials process and an example are illustrated in Figure 1. Patients who meet the strict criteria of a defined population are placed on study. The results

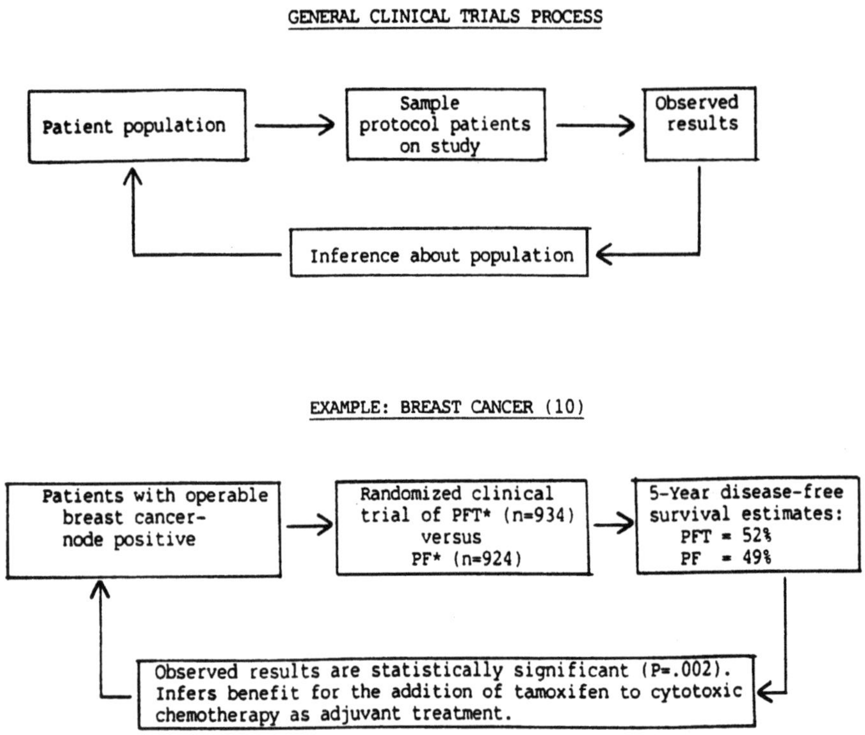

* PFT = L-phenylalanine mustard (L-PAM) + 5-fluorouracil (5-FU) + tamoxifen for two years of therapy

Figure 1. Clinical trials process

of the treatment of these patients are observed, and statistical evaluations of the data are performed. The results of these analyses are used as evidence to make inferences about how the treatment might be applied for the benefit of the larger population. In the example (10), patients with operable breast cancer and positive axillary node involvement are randomized, following mastectomy, to receive either combination chemotherapy with PF (L-phenylalanine mustard + 5-fluorouracil) or combined chemo-endocrine therapy with PF plus tamoxifen for 2 years (PFT). The observed results are summarized in terms of five year disease-free survival (DFS) estimates. It is important to distinguish these observed results (e.g., 52% DFS for the PFT treated group) from the effectiveness of treatment for the entire population. The observed results are used for the projected estimation of the DFS that would have been obtained if the entire population had been treated.

An observed treatment effect is composed of the following three elements:

Observed		Average		Random		Systematic
Treatment	=	Real	+	Error	+	Error
Effect		Effect		(Variability)		(Bias)

Systematic error (bias) refers to any feature that may cause the observed effect to be non-representative of the true effect that the trial is designed to estimate. Random error (variability) refers to the fact that a different sample of patients, even if selected in an identical manner from the same population, would yield a different observed result by chance alone. Bias and random chance will influence the results observed within any particular clinical trial, so that the observed treatment effect will not be exactly equal to the real treatment effect that is being estimated. As the goal of clinical trials is to obtain information about real treatment effect, the objectives of clinical trial methodology are, therefore, to:

1) minimize biases that might produce observed treatment effects which are distortions of the real impact of therapy,

and

2) minimize the variability of the trial estimates by evaluating an adequate sample size to detect treatment effects that might reasonably be expected.

REQUIREMENT OF STUDY DESIGN

The protocol document describes a complete plan for design and conduct of the clinical trial. The major components of the protocol are listed in Table 1. The list provides a guide to the main features which must be considered in clinical research.

REMARKS REGARDING THE PATIENT POPULATION

The definition of eligible patients must rely on conclusions drawn from existing data regarding the availability of 'effective' or 'ineffective' treatments. For example, sufficient data may be available to justify excluding patients with hormone receptor negative tumors from clinical trials which involve the evaluation of endocrine therapies. It is argued that including such patients in the trial may dilute our ability to detect treatment effects of the endocrine therapy by including a proportion of 'nonresponsive' patients in all treatment regimens. On the other hand, if the hormone receptor assay is not reliable, patients with true receptor positive tumors may be excluded, and the selection may change as the quality control of the laboratory changes. An alternative to excluding these patients would be to prospectively stratify the randomization and decide, before conducting the trial, that the results will be analyzed separately within patient subgroups defined by receptor status.

Table 1. Outline of protocol document.

Schema	- pictorial summary of the essentials of the study design. Should be simple and logical and reflecting the study objectives
Background	- prior results and rationale for the current study
Objectives	- few in number, relate to schema, feasible
Treatment allocation	- randomization to avoid bias, stratification to achieve balance, placebo control, cross-over plan etc.
Treatment	- give all details to describe administration schedule, potential toxicities, dose modification and duration
Follow-up procedures	- schedules, clinical and laboratory data
Endpoints	- standardize and quantify criteria for - evaluating treatment effects
Statistical considerations	- study design and sample size
Forms submission	- simple, efficient and comparable schedules for all treatment arms
Informed consent	- risks, benefits, alternative treatments (including no additional therapy) and right to withdraw

The variation in natural history of the disease for these patients is likely to be much larger than any observable differences in the effectiveness of treatment. Furthermore, the cutoff values for various features which may influence prognosis are not well established. Most of these factors influence prognosis along a continuum. For example, if a treatment is to be evaluated in 'high risk' patients, should those with four or more axillary lymph nodes involved be considered 'high risk'; or should ten or more positive nodes define 'high risk'?

Ideally, we would like to establish a study sample of patients with as homogeneous an outcome as possible. However, by attempting to define a homogeneous population for which maximum benefit might be achieved with minimal risks, we might find that too few patients are available to enter the protocol sample to meet the required accrual objectives. There is a trade-off between narrowly defining eligible patients and achieving sample size objectives.

REMARKS REGARDING THE ROLE OF RANDOMIZATION

Unfortunately, it is not possible to standardize and control all factors which might influence treatment outcome merely by careful definition in the protocol document. A fundamental priciple in experimental sciences for comparing two treatments is that groups must be alike in all aspects which are likely to affect outcome, so that any observed differences might be attributable only to the treatment applied or to random variation. Any systematic bias making the groups noncomparable may lead to observed differences in treatment effect when no real differences exist. Similarly, real treatment differences may be missed if the comparison groups are not comparable. The term randomization refers to the use of a chance mechanism as a means for allocating treatment to patients. By giving each patient the same opportunity to receive any of the therapies under investigation, the characteristics of the different groups will be 'alike on the average' with respect to all factors which are likely to affect outcome. In this way, any observed differences in results between groups will tend to be due to the treatment.

Any comparative analyses for which the groups are established by mechanisms other than randomization may be subject to patient selection biases and/or environmental system biases. The former refer to differences in natuaral history prognosis, and characteristics of the disease or patients which are likely to influence the outcomes of treatment. If the treatment groups differ with respect to these characteristics (e.g. number of axillary nodes involved), observed differences might be due to this imbalance rather than to any real effects to treatment. These kinds of biases may be partially controlled by stratification of the analysis, matching techniques, and mathematical modeling to compare treatment effects within more homogeneous subgroups of the patient population.

The environmental factor biases involve supportive care facilities, completeness of diagnostic work-up, aggressivity of treatment (philosophy of approach), training and experience of the surgeon, referral patterns, clinic waiting lists, quality and quantity of data collected, and any other feature characterizing the clinical setting of the investigation. These environmental biases cannot be corrected by sophisticated statistical modelling techniques and represent the major source of concern with respect to historically controlled analyses and analyses comparing treatment effects across studies. The biases due to environmental factors are largely nonquantifiable and therefore not amenable to corrective action. Only through prospective determination of control groups on the basis of some chance mechanism will these environmental factor biases be controlled 'on the average', making treatment comparisons unbiased within the trial.

We recognize that the use of randomization does not solve all of the difficulties in conducting clinical research trials for breast cancer. Treatment groups may still be unbalanced with respect to prognostic factors within a single study. Furthermore, randomization helps to establish internal validity only, but does nothing to insure that the protocol patients are representative of the larger population of interest. External validity, the appropriateness of extrapolating results from a clinical trial to the treatment of patients in standard clinical practice, is not established by randomization.

Several other techniques in addition to randomization are utilized to reduce the bias in comparisons of treatments. Often the randomization is stratified by factors which are felt to be prognostically important. Stratified randomization means that patients in different patient subpopulations are randomized separately so that an equal allocation of treatment to patients within a given stratum can be guaranteed. Stratified randomization provides a control against the chance occurrence of 'bad breaks' from the randomization, but in return adds an additional complexity to the treatment allocation process (11,12). Stratified randomization is also useful if possible treatment-host factor interactions are hypothesized. For example, if tamoxifen is being evaluated, prospective stratification by estrogen receptor status will allow separate analyses of treatment to be made for patients with ER positive and ER negative tumors that effectively can be considered as two separate concurrent randomized trials. This overcomes some of the problems with retrospective subgroup analyses, and avoids the dilution of effects from non-responsive patients that are mixed among those who respond.

Blinding is also used in the design of clinical trials to reduce biases of various types. Blinding refers to withholding information from the patient (single bind), patient and physician (double bind), or patient, physician and statistician (triple blind). The randomization is blinded so that physicians cannot select patients according to the treatment which will be allocated. Treatments are blinded so that any 'placebo effect' response will be balanced across the regimens. Blinding of the evaluation process means that the individual determinating the therapeutic response or examining the patient for possible recurrence is unaware of which treatment is being given. A recent study by the Eastern Cooperative Oncology Group (13) compared tamoxifen versus placebo as adjuvant for patients 66 to 80 years old. Blinding of the reports on early study results allows study entry and progress to continue without being prejudiced by premature and possibly unreliable impressions. For reasons of safety, only a study monitoring committee needs to be aware of the early results.

REMARKS REGARDING SAMPLE SIZE CONSIDERATIONS

Four entities must be specified in order to determine the sample size requirement for a comparative clinical trial. First, the criteria for measuring treatment difference must be specified and the test statistic which will be used to compare treatment outcomes must be given. For example, the logrank procedure is commonly used for comparing treatment outcomes based on relapse-free survival, overall survival, or other measures evaluating time to an event of interest. When recurrence or death (events) is the statistical endpoint of interest, statistical power is a function of the number of events observed rather than of the total number of patients entered.

The three remaining quantities (alpha, beta, delta) are shown in Table 2. Prospectively, for comparative study design purposes prior to obtaining any data, the table should be viewed within column, i.e. vertically. Alpha is the acceptable false positive

Table 2. The Decision-Truth Table

DECISION	TRUTH: The treatments have equal efficacy (H_0 is true)	TRUTH: The treatments have different efficacy by an amount Δ (H_0 is not true)
H_0 is true ($p > \alpha$)	O.K.	β-error Type II error
H_0 is not true ($p \leq \alpha$)	α-error Type I error	O.K. $1-\beta$ = power

α is usually set at 0.05
For design - view the table vertically
For analysis - view the table horizontally

rate of type I error. This is the probability of deciding, based on the observed data (our trial sample of the population), that there is a real treatment difference (for the entire population), when in fact no true treatment difference exists. Given that the correct answer is represented by the first column of the table, the mistake of deciding that there is a real treatment difference will be made only with the small probability of alpha. It has become standard practice to define alpha to be 0.05 or lower. This is two-sided if treatment differences in either direction would be considered worthy of reporting. For example, although a trial of adjuvant therapy versus a non-treatment control gorup would appear to represent a one-sided comparison (i.e., treatment is expected to improve outcome compared with no treatment), it may be possible for the treatment to have a deleterious effect. Only if such an unexpected negative outcome from the treatment results would never be interesting to report, is it reasonable to design the study as a one-sided comparison. Otherwise, sample sizes should be determined in order to provide adequate power to carry out two-sided tests of significance.

The quantities beta and delta are specified in the second column of the decision-truth table for the case when the treatment effects on the population are really different. Delta is the magnitude of this difference between treatment outcomes. Beta is the probability that we will fail to decide that there is a difference based on our clinical trial. This beta error is referred to as a type II error. When the true treatment difference for the population is delta, the probability of deciding based on our clinical trial that there is a difference between the treatment is 1-beta. This is called the statistical power of the test to detect treatment differences as large as delta. As the delta of clinical significance gets small, the statistical power to detect this difference in the clinical trial decreases. For a fixed value of delta, the power can be increased by increasing the number of events (e.g. patients who recur or die) within the sample. Therefore, given that a particular statistical endpoint and test procedure (e.g. logrank) will be used to evaluate treatment effects, the choices of alpha, beta and delta and anticipated underlying failure rates for the population of interest will determine the number of patients and events which are required to satisfy these criteria. For design purposes we set an accrual objective so that a clinically relevant difference (delta) will be detected with high probability (1-beta) when a decision rule designed to control alpha error (i.e. $p<0.05$) is used.

Table 3 shows the number of patients required to detect differences (delta) with probability 80% using a two-sided 0.05 level test for two examples; one for the adjuvant setting with survival as the endpoint of interest (14), and one for the advanced disease setting with response rate as the endpoint (15).

Therapeutic advances that are likely to be observed in the adjuvant setting require large numbers of patients and long periods of follow-up. Median survival of the control group might exceed 10 years. With 2 years of accrual and 3 additional years of follow-up, approximately 500 patients per treatment are required to detect a 50% improvement in median survival with a power of 80 using a 0.05 (two-sided) level test of statistical significance.

REMARKS REGARDING CONVENTIONAL AND QUALITY OF LIFE ORIENTED ENDPOINTS

Objective criteria need to be established as a measure of the impact of therapy. In studies involving patients with operable breast cancer, overall survival (OS) has been adopted as the ultimate criteria by which therapies are evaluated. Long follow-up periods are required in order to obtain good estimates of OS. Relapse-free survival (RFS) measures the time from operation to the recurrence of breast cancer. RFS has been assumed to be an early indicator of ultimate survival experience so that treatments providing improved RFS were considered to benefit the patient. Unfortunately, prolonged RFA has not resulted in improved OS within most of the adjuvant therapy trials reported to date. Substantially longer follow-up might be required before any difference in OS might be observed.

RFS provides an overly optimistic evaluation of the impact of therapy by considering patients who die without definitive evidence of breast cancer and those who develop a second malignancy as non-failures in the analysis (16). Some deaths without recurrence might be due to the treatment itself, and others may be found to have disease if autopsy had been performed. In order to reduce the overly optimistic evaluation of treatment effect, we recommend that disease-free survival (DFS) be reported in which patients who die are counted as failures (17).

A common error is made by reporting the distribution of site of first relapse considering only patients who failed as the denominator. The information gained from such an analysis is

Table 3. Examples for sample size requirements in an adjuvant and advanced disease setting

No of patients per treatment	Adjuvant Setting — Survival examples:[14] Lower median = 10 years, Accrual period= 2 years; Ratio of Medians: Additional Follow-up = 3 Years	Additional Follow-up = 7 Years	Advanced Disease — Response examples:[15] Lower Rate = 50% Difference in Rates
25	18.00	4.45	41%
50	4.40	2.65	29%
100	2.60	1.93	20%
200	1.90	1.58	14%
400	1.57	1.37	10%
600	1.44	1.29	8%

conditional on knowing prospectively which patients will relapse. A meaningful evaluation which reflects the impact of therapy upon patterns of relapse for the entire population should be made using the entire study sample as the denominator.

Not all sites of relapse have the same subsequent prognosis. While patients who have systemic failure are known to have a predictable dire prognosis, those with isolated mastectomy scar recurrence alone or those with operable cancer in the contralateral breast will have a less predictable outcome. Therefore, evaluation of systemic disease-free survival (SDFS) may provide a better indicator for ultimate overall survival than RFS (17).

Table 4 shows the five-year percentages at five years of median follow-up for the Ludwig III trial (18; see review of adjuvant therapy in this volume by Goldhirsch, Gelber, Mouridsen). The relative treatment effects on five possible conventional outcome measures for the group receiving chemo-endocrine therapy (CMFp+T) versus no adjuvant therapy (observation) are shown. The impact of treatment on relapse-free survival is over 2 1/4 times as large as the treatment difference in overall survival. Treatment decisions outside of trials will, therefore, depend upon the personal prejudice of the individual physician relying on the variety of endpoint measures to justify the choice of therapy.

Recently interest has increased in assessing treatment effectiveness based on quality-of-life oriented endpoints. Measurement of quality-of-life may be one of the most important considerations to infer the impact of therapy for the individual patient. The quality of one's life is a philosophical issue depending on the age of view, the treatment, the disease and the

Table 4. Treatment effect difference as evaluated by 5 different outcome measures: 5-year Kaplan-Meier rates LUDWIG III[18]

Endpoint Mesaure	Observation N=156	CMFp+T N=154	Odds Ratio CMFpT/OBS
Disease-free interval	32%	65%	3.9
Disease-free survival	31%	59%	3.2
Systemic disease-free survival	38%	60%	2.5
Survival (breast cancer deaths only)	61%	76%	2.0
Overall survival	59%	71%	1.7

environment in which the patient lives and in which the measurement is made. Performance status as assessed by the doctor in advanced disease applications restricts the patient's viewpoint and provides a somewhat objective measure of life quality. This assessment of functional status has been verified as a prognostic factor (19).

Other methods of measurement, such as the appearance of the patient to the physician or an expression by the patient regarding her own sense of well-being, are not readily reproducible and provide little standardization to enable extrapolation of the value of the measurement to other patients. The linear analogue self-assessment (LASA) is the most commonly used method for assessing some aspects concerning the quality of life for cancer patients (20). This technique is the basis for a Functional Living Index-Cancer (21) recently developed and validated. The prognostic utility of this index has yet to be determined. A simple statement from the patient (poor, moderate, good) about her perceived life quality may be sufficient to assess the impact of the therapy. As in melanoma (22), we may find that patients with breast cancer who claim they cope well with the disease are living longer. The psychological and social aspects involved with the diagnosis and treatment of breast cancer are far from being completely focused. The anxiety related to the diagnosis, the psychological morbidity of mastectomy, the role of adjuvant therapy and follow-up in reminding the patient of her disease are only some of the issues currently being investigated (23).

We have approached the problem of therapy selection from the quantitative rather than psychological point of view. The time without symptoms of disease and subjective toxic effects of adjuvant treatment (TWiST) is constructed by subtracting from overall survival those periods of time during which the patient is exposed to her disease or the subjective side effects of the adjuvant therapy. For this purpose we define a list of conditions for which time has been subtracted (Table 5).

Table 5. Construction of TWiST (Time Without Symptoms and Toxicity) for Individual Patients

Event	Time Removed from Total Survival
a. Leukopenia, thrombocytopenia and grade 1 or 2 anemia (asymptomatic)	No penalty
b. Any reversible subjective toxic effect of any grade (excluding amenorrhea) reported during a cycle or month of treatment	Remove the entire month
c. Alopecia and weight gain	Remove an additional three months after last report to allow for recovery
d. Isolated mastectomy scar or contralateral breast cancer alone	Remove three months to recovery from local procedure
e. Any appearance of relapse* (other than d.) or second primary tumor (not breast)	Remove entire remaining survival

* Skeletal recurrences were considered when symptomatic or at the initiation of systemic treatment.

This example of a quality of life endpoint is considered necessary to evaluate therapeutic benefit in a setting (adjuvant) in which all patients are initially exposed to toxic effects of treatment while a potential gain in overall survival might be experienced by some patients at a later time. The comparisons of CMFp+T versus observation and p+T (one year of low-dose prednisone plus tamoxifen) versus observation in the Ludwig III trial illustrate the utility of this new endpoint (Figure 2). The distributions of TWiST accumulated for treated patients are compared directly with the distributions of TWiST accumulated for patients in the observation group. Averaging these differences over the entire population of patients at each time from mastectomy provides values for the average net gain or loss of TWiST for treated patients compared with no adjuvant treatment. The substantial burden of early subjective toxic effects is compensated for by delay in subsequent exposure to disease so that by five years postmastectomy, a net gain is provided by either form of adjuvant therapy (Figure 2). The gain in TWiST for the chemo-endocrine regimen is larger and more rapidly increasing than the gain provided by the endocrine therapy alone.

TWiST analysis is the way to select adjuvant treatment until studies are mature enough to provide objective evidence for a survival advantage (24,25).

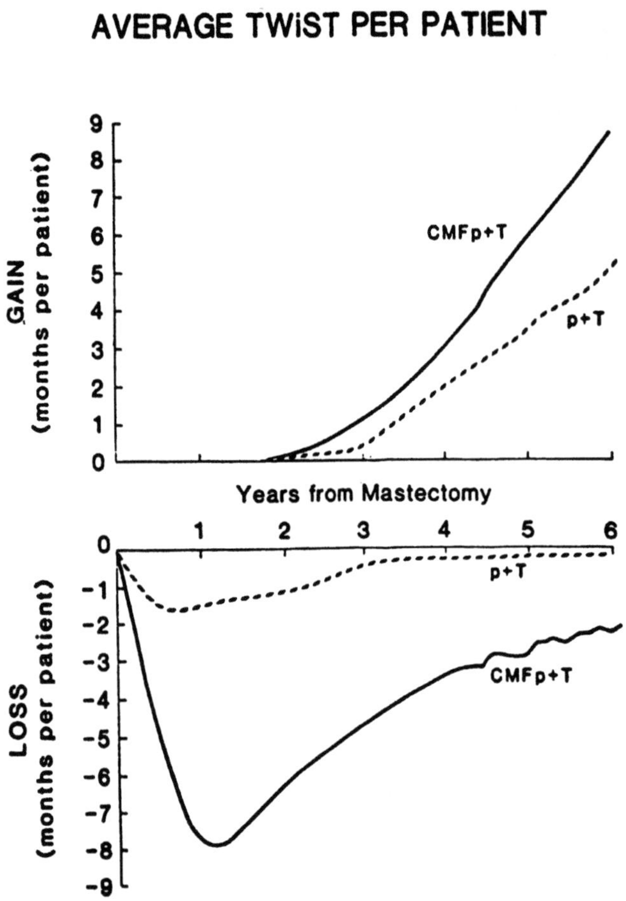

Fig. 2. Average TWiST gained or lost per treated patient as functions of time (T) from mastectomy. CMFp+T vs observation (solid lines) and p+T vs observation (dashed lines).

STATISTICAL PROOF: WHAT DOES IT MEAN?

Many investigators take the results of clinical trials as representing a proof of a hypothesis of interest. Table 2 when considered horizontally represents the decision-making criteria applied at the time of data analysis. The standard way of evaluating statistical evidence is to compute a p-value which indicates the probability of obtaining the observed treatment differences (plus differences more extreme than those observed), if we pretend that the treatments really have equivalent effects when given to the total population. The usual convention is to consider $p \leq 0.05$ as an indication that the treatment may not produce equivalent effects. The rationale for this interpretation is that p-values $p \leq 0.05$ occur only rarely by chance alone. If $p \leq 0.05$, then we decide that the treatments are different as indicated by the bottom row in Table 2. It is possible that the treatments have identical therapeutic effects (the first column of Table 2), and that we, in fact, observed a rare event. Thus, obtaining $p \leq 0.05$ does not prove that the treatments have different effects. Similarly, if we obtain $p > 0.05$ (top row of

Table 2), it is possible that the treatments really have effects which differ by an amount delta (second column of Table 2), but that our trial failed to detect this difference due to a high beta error. Thus failure to demonstrate a statistically significant difference also does not prove that the treatments really have equivalent effects. Therefore, conducting a well-designed clinical trial can only provide convincing evidence for or against treatment differences, but does not represent proof on a clearly black or white basis.

INTERPRETATION AND CONCLUSIONS FROM ANALYSES OF SUBGROUPS: ENDOCRINE MECHANISMS

A common practice is to devote a large part of a report on clinical trials to the analysis of treatment effects within various subgroups of the patients in the study. This is particularly true for studies involving investigations of endocrine mechanisms. Some patients are assumed to have hormone-dependent disease while others are assumed to have hormone-independent tumors. It only remains to accurately classify patient subgroups in order to determine who will and who will not respond to endocrine therapy. Two difficulties for achieving this objective are:

i) inability to prospectively identify patients who might respond,

and

ii) problems with the retrospective analysis of treatment effects within subgroups.

From the perspective of designing trials, one must separate the role of stratification for identifying patient subgroups having different prognoses, from the role of stratification for the purpose of distinguishing patients who are likely to respond from those who are likely to be non-responsive to therapy (see Role of randomization). It is important to distinguish between the notion of differences in baseline prognoses, and the notion of differences in degree of improvement under treatment. The role of stratification in the first case is to achieve balance between treatment groups with respect to baseline prognoses, so that observed differences in outcome might be entirely attributed to the effects of therapy. Stratification in the second case provides a prospective basis for separate analyses and testing of hypotheses by subgroups.

Retrospective analyses of treatment effects within multiple subgroups have an increased likelihood of finding a false positive effect by virtue of the multiplicity of analyses. If the data analysis within each subgroup has a 5% possibility to achieve statistical significance by chance alone, the chance of finding at least one significant result within some subgroup is much greater than the nominal value of 5%. In addition, multiple subgroup analyses increase the chance that a spurious treatment-subgroup interaction effect might be indicated. Therefore, when such effects are found in the data, we should report the findings, but not believe them (26).

The investigator's desire to evaluate treatment effects within subgroups of the patient population is a manifestation of this desire to treat the individual patient with the best available regimen designed specifically for the individual. This desire is in conflict with the main research capabilities of the clinical trial. Unfortunately, analyses of patient subgroups within a clinical trial have a high risk of producing false positive results. Furthermore, subdividing the patient population will result in too few patients remaining for analysis in any specific subgroup. Finally, if the results of subgroup analyses are taken incorrectly as 'statistical proof' of a treatment effect, physicians may find it difficult to withhold apparently effective treatment, and the reconfirmation of the initial findings may become impossible. Subgroup analyses of clinical trial data should be performed to generate research hypotheses and to gain insights regarding the possible mechanism of action of therapies. However, such analyses should not be used to tailor-make treatment for the individual patient without reconfirmation of findings from additional sources, even if the results are in agreement with a pet hypotesis of the investigators. The results from the overall study population should remain the major component of the report on a treatment advance.

Drug interaction refers to synergism or antagonism that is seen with a combination of two or more agents, which would not occur

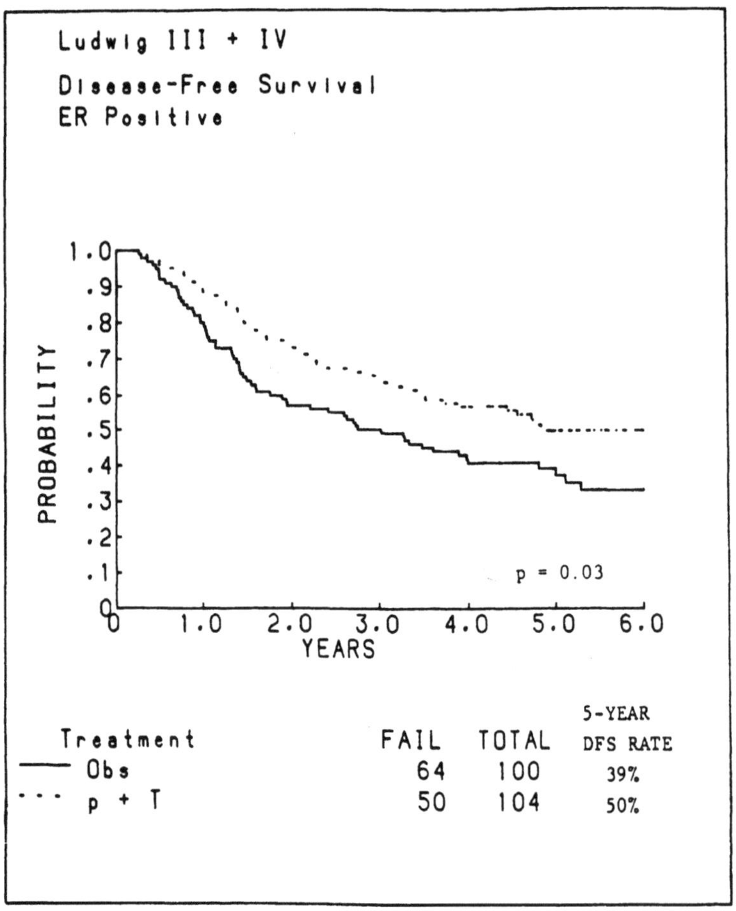

Fig. 3.
Disease-free survival by Treatment for Ludwig Studies III and IV at 5 years median follow-up

Fig. 3A
All patients

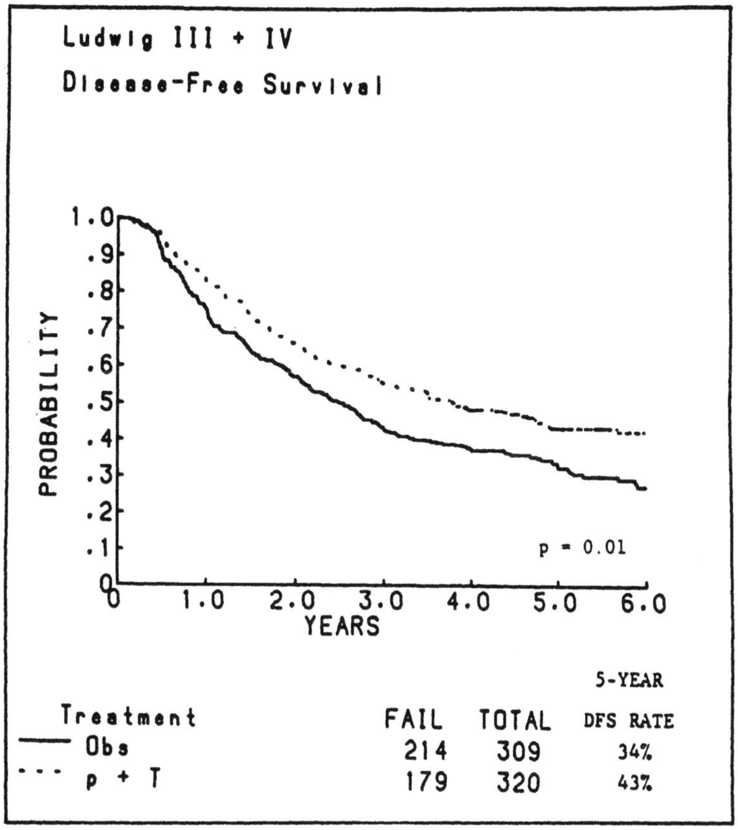

Fig. 3B Patients with estrogen receptor positive tumors (≥ 10 fmol/mg cytosol protein)

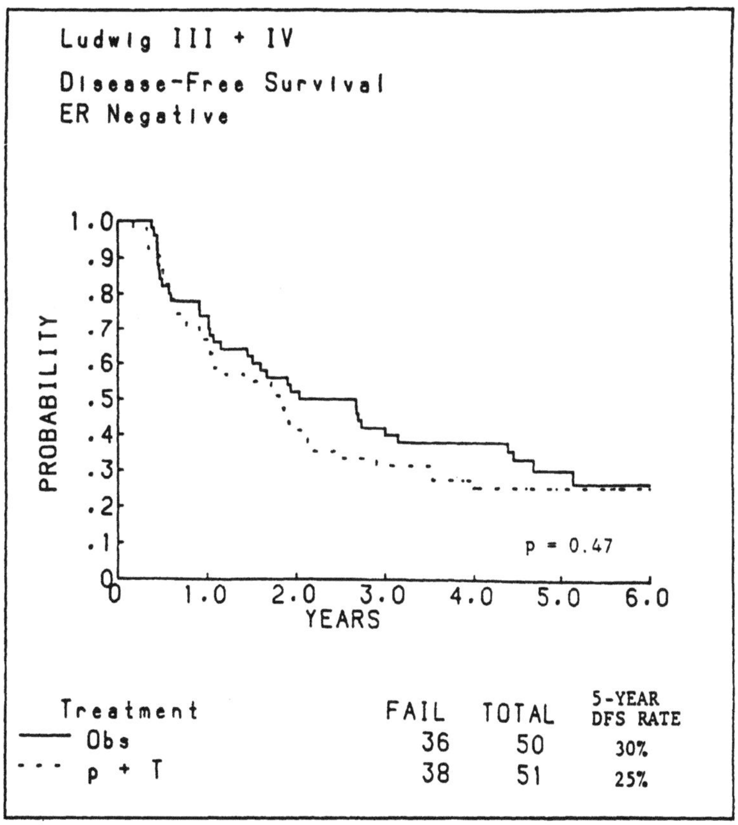

Fig. 3C Patients with estrogen receptor negative tumors (0-9 fmol/mg cytosol protein)

with either agent separately. Statistical interaction between treatment and patient subset exists if the effectiveness of the therapy is different for different subsets of patients.
An interaction is present in a treatment comparison if the differences in therapeutic outcome are different for different groups of patients. These interactions are roughly defined as quantitative if the magnitude, but not the direction, of the effects is different (differences in degree), while qualitative interactions are those for which the direction of the effects is different (difference in kind). Quantitative interactions are quite common, while qualitative interactions are are. The study of endocrine treatments for breast cancer probably represents one of the areas for which qualitative interactions are not so rare. The role of estrogen receptor and progesterone receptor content in the primary tumor for identifyng possible treatment-subgroup interactions is an example.

Results from the Ludwig Trials III + IV (27; see adjuvant therapy review in this volume) comparing endocrine adjuvant therapy with low-dose prednisone and tamoxifen versus observation in postmenopausal patients with positive axillary node metastases are shown in Figure 3A. The analysis of DFS at 5 years median follow-up indicates an advantage for the p+T treated group. 48% of the patients had estrogen receptor content of the primary determined, with approximately one-third of these classified as negative (less than 10 fmol/mg cytosol protein).

The analysis of treatment effects by subgroups suggests that the impact of p+T is confined to patients with positive estrogen receptor tumors (p=0.03, Figure 3B); p+T is not effective for patients with ER negative tumors (p=0.47, Figure 3C). However, the statistical test for a quantitative interaction is not significant (p=0.20). Nevertheless, we might be tempted to believe our pet hypothesis that endocrine therapy is effective only in patients with tumors which contain higher amounts of estrogen receptors.

Consider, however, the example of outcome for Ludwig II by receptor status, for premenopausal patients with four or more axillary node metastases (28; see adjuvant therapy review in this volume). In this case, an unexpected benefit is observed for the oophorectomy plus CMFp group compared with CMFp alone, but only among patients with PgR negative tumors (Figure 4A). In the same study, some evidence is emerging to suggest a late, but as yet not statistically significant benefit for the combined modality regimen among patients with ER positive tumors (Figure 4B). As suggested by Peto (26), we might report the first result, but do not believe it; while the second result might suggest some chance for optimism in the future. Both results, however, need clinical verification which must be based on prospective and not retrospective evaluation.

A careful attempt to define a proper statistical method of testing for qualitative interactions between treatment effects and patient subgroups has been recently published (29). The method was applied to the results of the NSABP trial B-09 which compares a 5-fluorouracil-melphalen combination (PF) with the same combination plus tamoxifen (PFT) (10). While the test did not demonstrate a statistically significant qualitative

Fig. 4. Disease-free sur- vival by treatment for Ludwig Study II at 5 years median follow-up

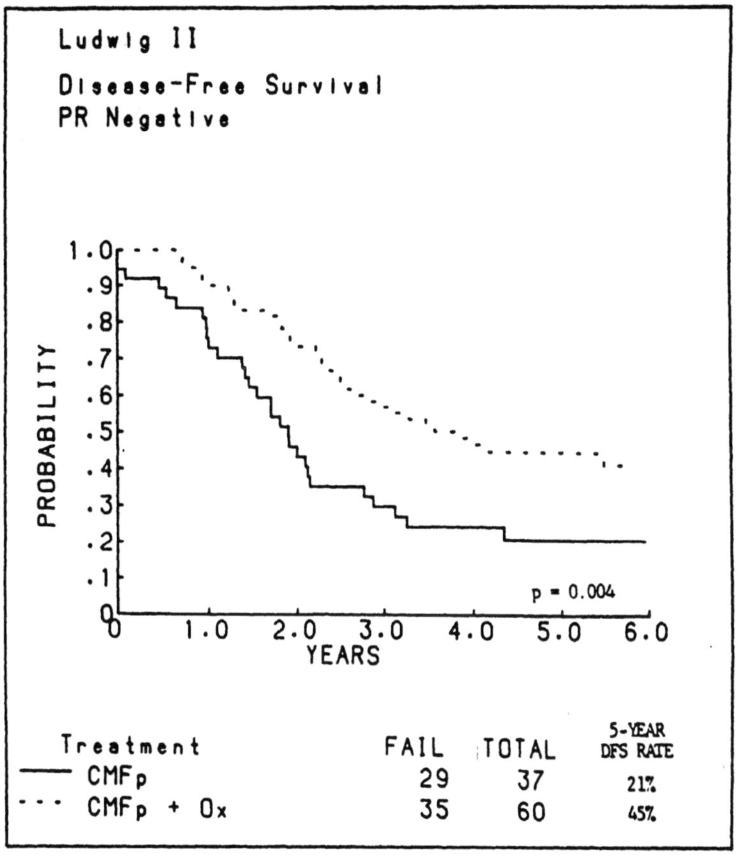

Fig. 4A Patients with progesterone receptor negative tumors (0-9 fmol/mg cytosol protein)

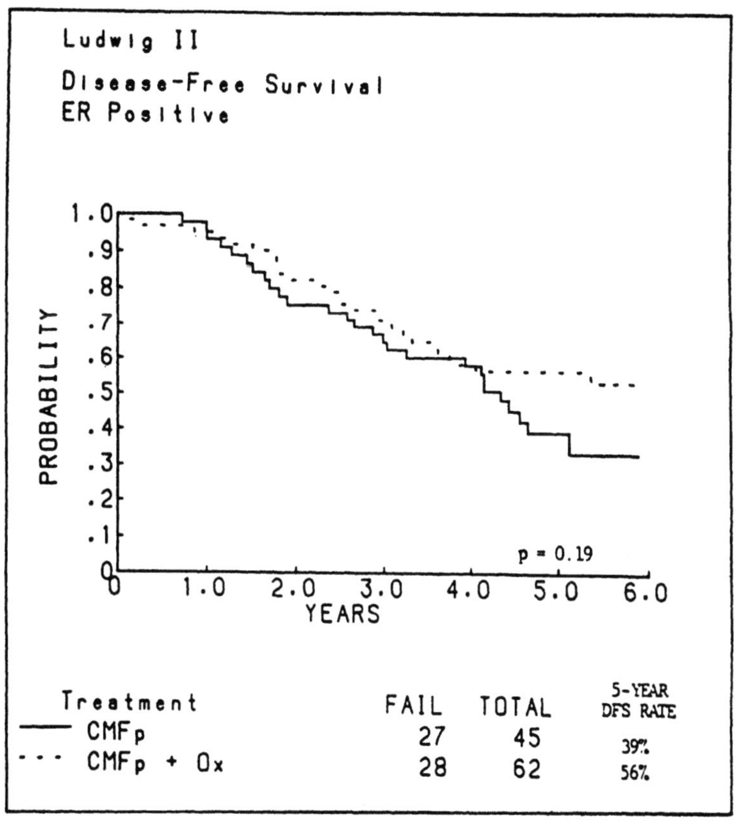

Fig. 4B Patients with estrogen receptor positive tumors (≥ fmol/mg cytosol protein)

interaction between treatments and subgroups defined by age and PgR content of the primary, it is important to note that the statistical power for the test is remarkably low. Furthermore, the demonstration of a qualitative interaction might be too restrictive as a prerequisite for adopting different clinical practice for different subpopulations. Subgroup effects that are quantitatively different (i.e., small positive effect for one group, large positive effect for another) may be sufficient especially in view of toxic side effects and other costs of treatment.

REMARKS CONCERNING OVERVIEW PROCEDURES = META-ANALYSIS

Meta-analysis of randomized clinical trials is an attempt to derive from all available trials a summary of results concerning the endpoint which is a common feature of all the studies. The conduct of such an exercise is itself a clinical trial and requires:

1. International cooperation (all eligible and appropriate trials included),

2. Selection of trials which are quality controlled with respect to their patient population, treatments, compliance, endpoint etc.,

   and

3. Careful interpretation and recognition of strenghts and weaknesses.

The main strength of an overview is to properly accumulate evidence from many trials in order to detect treatment effects that are too small to be found in the individual studies alone. The main weakness of an overview is the tendency to obscure the differences between studies being combined and to perform indirect comparisons between trials that ask different questions (30,31).

Two recent overviews of trials were conducted to evaluate the impact on overall survival of adjuvant therapy for breast cancer (32). All randomized trials that compared tamoxifen versus nil, or tamoxifen plus other therapy versus the other therapy alone were used to estimate the effectiveness of the endocrine therapy. A concomitant overview was conducted for trials involving the use of chemotherapy as adjuvant treatment. The tendency to compare the results of these two overviews, especially in postmenopausal patients, has led many to conclude that endocrine therapy is superior to chemotherapy, despite the fact that a direct comparison between these modalities has not been extensively performed. In addition, comparison of results from a subgroup of studies within an overview versus results from a different subgroup of studies (e.g., those using one year of tamoxifen versus those using two or more years of tamoxifen) has been interpreted as providing indirect evidence for the superiority of the prolonged administration. This conclusion, despite its agreement with a pet hypothesis, requires a prospective confirmation from a randomized trial or from an overview of trials, all of which address this specific question.

SPECIAL FEATURES OF TRIALS IN THE ADJUVANT SETTING

Some special aspects of adjuvant treatment influence the methodological requirements for clinical trials (Table 6).

In spite of surgery for the primary tumor that renders the patient clinically free of disease, the likelihood of recurrence

Table 6. Adjuvant Setting: Special Features and Their Methodological Consequences

Feature	Consequence
1. Curative intent of treatment; patient is objectively free of disease	- Limitation regarding acceptable toxicity (early and late) of treatment.
2. Heterogeneous population	- Randomized comparison required. - Proper stratification and identification of subgroups (e.g. markers of endocrine dependency).
3. Low annual failure rate	- Large sample size and long follow-up periods are required. - Improvements can be seen in a small proportion of patients (concept of avoidable events).
4. Continual failure rate	- Treatment impact may be detected later (after a long follow-up period).
5. Small treatment effects	- Large number of patients and an overview of trials are needed.
6. Treatment effects appear at different times (chemotherapy after short follow-up; and endocrine therapy after longer follow-up)	- Consideration of follow-up maturity is required. - Identification of prognostic feature only after a long period of follow-up.

and eventual death due to breast cancer still exists for most patients. In contrast to the advanced disease setting, however, treatment is given with a curative as opposed to a palliative intent. Special features of the patients, their disease, and its treatment complicate the objectives of proper methodology in the adjuvant setting. These include the heterogeneity of the population, the relatively low failure rate, the continual rate of failure over time, small effects of currently availabe adjuvant therapies, and late appearing differences. The fact that ultimate prognosis for an individual patient is unpredictable and that the stakes are high represent the main considerations concerning methodological issues.

The heterogeneity of the population with respect to outcome is illustrated by the variety of end results predictable based on an assessment of axillary nodal status at the time of operation. Patients with no axillary node involvement have a 5-year survival rate exceeding 85%, while those with axillary node involvement have a 5-year survival percentage of 60%. A variety of other factors have been suggested to predict outcome in the adjuvant setting. These include patient-related features (age, menopausal status, body mass, family history) and tumor-related features (tumor size, hormone receptor status, labelling index, ploidy of tumor cells, vascular invasion, tumor grade, tumor type). Although the importance of each of these factors relative to each other, the magnitude of their predictive ability, the independence of each to the other, and the description of the causative versus the associative relationships have yet to be determined, it is clear that the ability to predict outcome in an individual patient is extremely difficult. This heterogeneity of outcome places a large burden on the clinical trial to control for the additional variability associated with the estimation of treatment effects. The heterogeneity of patient outcome makes it difficult to know to what extent observed results are due to real treatment effects as opposed to selection of patients destined to have a more favorable outcome. In a comparative trial, groups being compared must be alike with respect to all features that might influence outcome. This is exclusively achieved by randomization. Only in this way can any differences between the groups be attributed to the treatment effect, especially if small (as expected in the adjuvant setting).

In the adjuvant setting, relapse and death due to breast cancer treated with local means alone occur in a relatively low proportion of patients per annum and at a rather steady rate. Presumably this is particularly true for patients whose tumors contain higher concentrations of hormone receptors. A large sample size and long periods of follow-up are required in order to observe a sufficiently high number of failures to obtain acceptable statistical power. Because only patients who would otherwise relapse can benefit from adjuvant therapy, the fewer patients who might relapse the fewer there are who could benefit. The concept of avoidable relapse is important for judging the value of an adjuvant treatment program for a relatively good risk population.

The size of effects reported for currently available adjuvant therapies is small, making the detection of these effects difficult. Large sample sizes in individual trials and an overview of all available randomized trials are required. Furthermore, and most relevant for endocrine therapy, is the suggestion that the magnitude of the treatment effects might be different at different times during the course of follow-up of the patients. Data suggest that the effect of chemotherapy during a short period after mastectomy is to delay recurrences. This might be an explanation for the striking results in favor of chemotherapy in the late seventies. On the other hand, during the initial period postmastectomy endocrine therapy appears to reduce the incidence of those recurrences which are indicators for a better post-relapse survival outcome (i.e., local and local/regional). The overall survival differences, therefore, in trials evaluating endocrine therapies are to be expected to emerge only after a longer period of follow up.

Failure to detect significant treatment effects in early reports of these trials investigating endocrine mechanisms is not surprising.

SPECIAL FEATURES OF TRIALS IN THE ADVANCED DISEASE SETTING

Once the patient relapses, with very few exceptions (e.g., isolated local recurrence, contralateral breast cancer) the fact that the disease clinically appeared or reappeared is related to a dire prognosis. The great majority of patients with this stage of disease will die of breast cancer. The features of the disease at this stage which might influence the conduct and interpretation of results of clinical trials are described in Table 7.

The prognosis of patients with advanced disease is related to a variety of indicators which distinguish both the baseline prognosis and responsiveness to palliative treatment. These include organ sites of metastatic involvement, performance status, preceding tumor free interval, steroid hormone receptor content, response to prior therapy, etc. A wide range of outcomes in terms of duration of future survival time is a consequence of these characteristics. The conduct of trials separately within each one of these subpopulations defined by so-called "good" or "bad" prognostic factors might provide information about real treatment effectiveness that might be obscured in a study that includes all ranges of prognosis. This is especially true because the expected improvements with treatment for each one of the subgroups is likely to be small. For example, premenopausal patients with multiple organ involvement are likely to have a disease which is refractory to endocrine manipulations. On the other hand, response and subsequent palliation may be achieved with hormonal therapy for patients with tissue metastasis or with bony disease alone.

Furthermore, the anticipated survival for these two groups is so different that an improvement in the "good" risk group might be completely obscured by early deaths among the "poor" risk subgroup. The evaluation of endocrine therapy in a sample of patients that includes both subgroups will, therefore, be diluted (33).

Table 7. Advanced disease setting: Special features and their methodological consequences

Feature	Consequence
1. Palliative intent of therapy	- Response rate determination with survival and with some indication for quality of life.
2. Imprecise measurement of response	- Difficult interpretation and extrapolation of study resuts.
3. Existence of multiple prognostic factors (site dependent, performance status dependent, etc.)	- Need for separate studies based on prognostic subgroup
4. Response to first treatment predicts the response to the subsequent therapy (especially for therapy for endocrine manipulations).	- Evaluation of secondary treatment (e.g.cross-over) must be conducted separately for each
Resistance to first therapy predicts resistance to subsequent therapy.	first-therapy-response group.
5. Responders live longer than nonresponders	- Feature of the disease and its evaluation that do not necessarily indicate a treatment advantage

Measuring response treatment of advance disease is an area of controversy and represents a methodological obstacle especially for design of studies for determination of activity of new agents. The special features of definition of response will be the theme of a future discussion within the framework of this Task Force.

It is, however, important to consider an important methodological issue concerning investigation of the anti-neoplastic activity of endocrine agents in advanced breast cancer. These methodological issues are derived from the fact that the response to a previous endocrine manipulation is a major predictor of response to a secondary hormonal therapy. On the other hand, primary progressive disease under hormonal therapy almost always predicts no response for subsequent endocrine manipulation. Since evidence exists about the fact that combination endocrine therapy does not carry an additional advantage when compared with a treatment using a single endocrine agent, the objective for actual trials remains the optimization of sequential use of endocrine agents (see review of advanced disease in this volume by Mouridsen).

Randomized trials of primary endocrine therapies (e.g., oophorectomy versus tamoxifen in premenopausal patients) with subsequent cross-over represent important examples for sample size issues concerning the activity of each one of these endocrine therapies as secondary intervention after the other. The sample size consideration is illustrated in Figure 5.

Table 3 indicates that 100 patients per group is an adequate sample size to detect a 20% improvement in response rate between two forms of endocrine therapy. However, because only the responders to the initial agent are likely to respond to the cross-over, only a fraction of the original sample (approximately 30%) will be available for evaluation of the question of sequential utility of the agents. The response to the initial agent effectively stratifies the evaluation of the cross-over efficacy into two separate studies. Clinical trials investigating endocrine mechanisms in advanced disease require substantially more patients than are usually included in such trials.

SPECIAL FEATURES OF TRIALS IN THE PREVENTION SETTING

Prevention of breast cancer, or at least delaying its emergence until much later in life, may be the most effective way to reduce the mortality from the disease. Strategies involve either primary prevention (altering risk factors to reduce the likelihood of developing the disease), or secondary prevention (early detection of the disease at a stage which is more responsive to available therapies).

There are numerous methodological issues concerning studies of secondary prevention methods and the interpretation of results (34,35). These include length-biased sampling (by which more indolent pre-clinical disease is likely to be detected in a screening program), and lead-time bias (by which longer survival time is due in part to starting the clock earlier). Studies of scree-

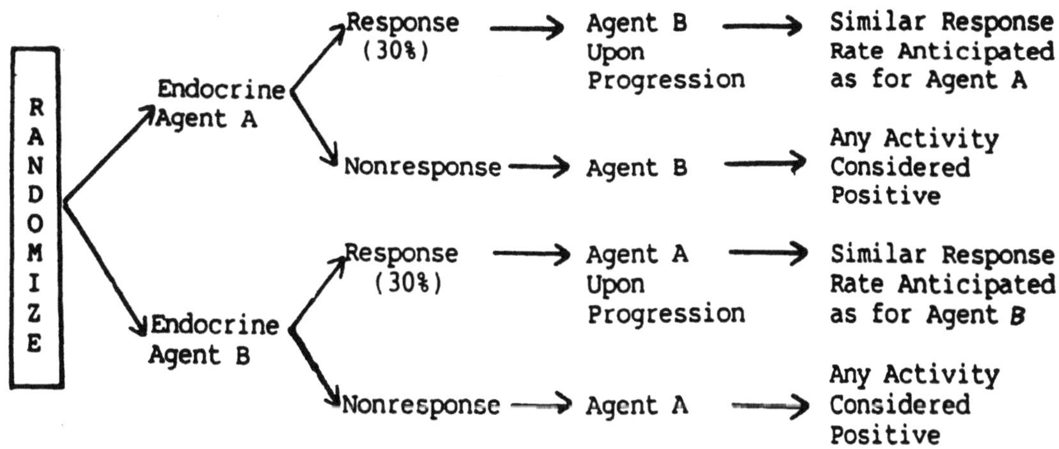

Figure 5. Randomized crossover design evaluating sequential use of endocrine agents A and B.

ning programs must adjust for these biases by establishing appropriate control groups and applying methods to provide unbiased analyses.

Primary prevention strategies can involve a variety of interventions ranging from motion of behavioral habits (e.g. changes in diet), preventive surgery (e.g. prophylactic mastectomy), to active long-term medical treatment (e.g., chemoprevention). Recent interest has developed regarding the use of tamoxifen as a chemoprevention agent to inhibit the development of breast cancer (see review of prevention issues by Jordan in this volume). Special features of primary prevention of breast cancer and their methodologic implications are described in Table 8 (36).

Because the incidence of the endpoint event of interest, development of breast cancer, is very low in the normal population, very large sample sizes (5,000-10,000 wowen) are required. Sample sizes must also account for the possibility of a high "drop-out" rate where healthy subjects elect to discontinue long-term use of the study agent. A "drop-in" phenomenon must also be considered in which subjects in the control group seek active treatment in violation of the assignment. "Drop-out" and "drop-in" are particularly troublesome for prevention trials due to the long periods of time the interventions must be maintained.

In order to increase the chance of detecting prevention effects, selection of study subjects must be restricted to "high-risk" populations. This not only increases the baseline incidence rate that might be effected, but also reduces the dilution due to competing (non-breast cancer) causes of failure among the study

Table 8. Prevention of Breast Cancer: Special Features and Their Methodological Consequences

Features	Consequence
1. Incidence of breast cancer in a normal population is low	- Accurate determination of high risk subset is essential.
2. Occurence of other malignancies and additional competing risks	- Sample size and age chosen to account for these events. (low-age high breast cancer risk population).
3. Therapy not clearly without long-term risk	- Adequate studies of toxic effects are required. - Potential for overtreatment. - Consider other ways of prevention: screening, dietary intervention, etc.

patients. Selection of a "high-risk" population also creates opportunity to yield a more favorable benefit to risk ratio.

The potential benefit of a prevention program is measured not only in terms of reduction of breast cancer incidence, but also in terms of the amount of lifetime gained without exposure to the diagnosis of breast cancer. Older populations of women have less to gain in this respect, and also experience a high incidence of competing causes of failure. Prevention trials in older women may provide little real benefit.

Younger women have a greater time at risk for developing breast cancer and a lower incidence of competing failures. A "high-risk" population of young women would have the most to gain from an effective prevention program. Unfortunately, these women also have the most to lose from unforeseen late toxic effects of chemoprevention interventions. This is especially true for therapies that influence endocrine function in premenopausal women.

Extreme caution must be used for investigating prevention strategies with unknown late sequelae. Selection of subjects must be restricted to those at highest risk who have the most to gain, even if this conflicts with the requirement to have a very large sample size. Cooperation across a wide geographical area is required. Attention should continue on studies of less invasive measures such as dietary recommendations and screening programs. The long-term risks of chemoprevention must be better understood before large scale studies designed to investigate benefit are undertaken.

REFERENCES

1. Mike' V: Clinical studies in cancer: a historical perspective. In: Mike' V, Stanley KE (eds). Statistics in Medical Research. New York: Wiley 1982 :111-155
2. Pocock SJ: Clinical Trials: A pratical approach. Chichester: John Wiley 1983
3. Buyse ME, Staquet MJ and Sylvester RJ (eds): Cancer Clinical Trials: Methods and Practice. Oxford: Oxford University Press 1984
4. Mike' V and Stanley KE (eds): Statistics in medical research: methods and issues, with applications in cancer research. New York: John Wiley and Sons 1982
5. Friedman LM, Furberg CD and DeMets DL: Fundamental of Clinical Trials. Boston: John Wright-PSG Inc 1982
6. Shapiro SH and Louis TA (eds) Clinical trials: issues and approaches. New York: Marcel Dekker Inc 1983
7. Bonadonna G and Valagussa P: Adjuvant systemic therapy for resectable breast cancer. J Clin Oncol 1985 (3):259-275
8. Goldhirsch A, Gelber RD, Davis BW: Adjuvant chemotherapy trials in breast cancer: an appraisal and lessons for patient care outside the trials. In: Forbes JF (ed) Clinical Surgery International. Vol 10 Breast disease. Edinburgh: Churchill Livingstone 1985:128-138
9. Henderson IC and Canellos GP: Cancer of the breast: The past decade. N Engl J of Med 1980 (302):17-30 and 78-90

10. Fisher B, Redmond C, Brown A, Fisher ER, Wolmark N, Bowan D, Plotkin D, Wolter J, Bornstein R, Legault-Poisson S, Saffer EA and other NSABP Investigators: Adjuvant chemotherapy with and without tamoxifen in the treatment of primary breast cancer: 5-year results from the National Surgical Adjuvant Breast and Bowel Project trial. J Clin Oncol 1986 (4):459-471
11. Zelen M: The randomization and stratification of patients to clinical trials. J Chron Diseases 1974 (27):365-375
12. Peto R, Pike MC, Armitage P et al: Design and analysis of clinical trials requiring prolonged observation of each patient. Br J Cancer 1977 part I (34):585-612 and part II (35):1-39
13. Cummings FJ, Gray R, Davis TE, Tormey DC, Harris JE, Falkon G and Arseneau J: Adjuvant tamoxifen treatment of elderly women with stage II breast cancer. Ann Int Med 1985 (103):324-329
14. Lesser ML and Cento SJ: Tables of power for the F-test for comparing two exponential survival distributions. J Chron Diseases 1981 (34):533-544
15. Fleiss JL: Statistical methods for rates and proportions. New York: John Wiley and Sons 1981: 38-48, 260-280
16. Kay R and Schumacher M: Unbiased assessment of treatment effects on disease recurrence and survival in clinical trials. Statistics in Medicine 1983 (2):41-59
17. Ludwig Breast Cancer Study Group. Randomized trial of chemo-endocrine therapy, endocrine therapy and mastectomy a-lone in postmenopausal patients with operable breast cancer and axillary node metastasis. Lancet 1984 (1):1256-1260
18. Goldhirsch A: Adjuvant therapy for postmenopausal women with operable breast cancer: Part I - a randomized trial of chemo-endocrine versus endocrine therapy versus mastectomy alone. In: Jones SE and Salomon SE (eds) Adjuvant therapy of cancer IV. Orlando: Grune and Stratton 1984: 379-391
19. Yates JW, Chalmer B, McKegney FP: Evaluation of patients with advanced cancer using the Karnofsky Performance Status. Cancer 1980 (45):2220-2224
20. Coates A, Fischer-Dillenbeck C, McNeil DR et al: On the receiving end II. Linear analogue self-assessment (LASA) in evaluation of aspects quality of life of cancer patients receiving therapy. Europ J Cancer and Clin Oncol 1983 (19):1633-1637
21. Schipper H, Clinch J, McMurray A, Levitt M: Measuring the quality of life of cancer patients. The functional living index-cancer development and validation. J Clin Oncol 1984 (2):472-483
22. Rogentine GN, Van Kammen DP, Fox BH et al: Psychological factors in the prognosis of malignant melanoma: a prospective study. Psychosomatic Medicine 1979 (4) (8):647-655
23. Maguire P and Van Dam F: Psycological aspects of breast cancer workshop report. Europ J Cancer and Clin Oncol 1983 (19):1735-1740
24. Gelber RD and Goldhirsch A: Adjuvant therapy in operable breast cancer: A definition of benefit (abstract) Controlled clinical trials 1985 (6):226
25. Gelber RD and Goldhirsch A: A new endpoint for the assessment of adjuvant therapy in postmenopausal women with operable breast cancer. (submitted).

26. Peto R: Statistical aspects of cancer trials. In: Halnan KE (ed) Treatment of Cancer. London: Chapman and Hall 1982: 867-871
27. Gelber RD: Adjuvant therapy for postmenopausal women with operable breast cancer: Part II - randomized trials comparing endocrine therapy with surgery alone. In: Jones SE and Salmon SE (eds) Adjuvant therapy of Cancer IV. Orlando: Grune and Stratton 1984: 393-406
28. Ludwig Breast Cancer Study Group. Chemotherapy with or without oophorectomy in high-risk premenopausal patients with operable breast cancer. J Clin Oncol 1985 (3):1059-1067
29. Gail M and Simon R: Testing for qualitative interactions between treatment effects and patient subsets. Biometrics 1985 (41):361-372
30. Carter SK: Interpretation of results of chemotherapy trials in breast cancer. J Clin Oncol 1986 (4):260-261
31. Gelber RD and Goldhirsch A: The concept of an overview of clinical trials in breast cancer (submitted).
32. UK-BCTS/UICC/WHO: Review of mortality results in randomized trials in early breast cancer. Lancet 1984 (2):1205
33. Cavalli F, Goldhirsch A snd Senn HJ: Interpretation of results of chemotherapy trials in metastatic breast cancer. J Clin Oncol 1986 (4):260-261
34. Milbrath JR, Moskowitz M and Bauermeister D: Breast cancer screening. In: CRC Critical Reviews in Diagnostic Imaging 1981: 181-218
35. Zelen M: Theory of early detection of breast cancer in the general population. In: Heuson JC, Mattheim WH and Rozencweig M (eds) Breast Cancer: Trends in Research and Treatment. New York: Raven Press 1976:287-302
36. Sestili MA and Dell JG (eds): Chemoprevention clinical trials: problems and solutions, 1984. Proceedings of a workshop, May 17-18, 1984. NIH Publication 1984 n.85-2715

Endocrine Treatment of Advanced Breast Cancer

H. T. Mouridsen

Department of Oncology ONA, The Finsen Institute, 49 Strandboulevarden, Copenhagen, Denmark

The various endocrine therapies available in the treatment of breast cancer can be divided into four groups according to their demonstrated or suggested mode of biological action (table 1). These include ablative therapy, inhibitive therapy, additive therapy and competitive therapy.

The rationale for the use of the ablative procedures is that hormones promote the growth of some mammary tumor cells. Thus a decrease in the concentration of these hormones is assumed to induce tumor regression (1-5).

The mechanism of action of aminoglutethimide has recently been described in detail (6). Briefly, it inhibits the production of the adrenal steroid hormones and the peripheral aromatization of androstenedione to estrone. Similar mechanisms of action have been described for the synthetic steroid trilostane (7). The mechanisms of action of danazol, a synthetic testosterone derivative, probably include binding to progesterone and androgen receptors (8) and inhibition of the steroid synthesis in the ovaries as well (9,10). The LH-RH analogues lead to a striking fall in plasma sex steroids via interference with the secretion of hypophyseal peptides (11).

The mode of action underlying the paradoxical effect of pharmacological doses of steroid hormones such as estrogens,

Table 1. Endocrine therapy of advanced breast cancer.

Ablative	Oophorectomy Adrenalectomy Hypophysectomy
Additive	Estrogen Progestin Androgen
Competitive	Antiestrogen
Inhibitive	Aminoglutethimide Trilostane Danazol LH-RH analogues

androgens, progestins and glucocorticoids on tumor growth is largely unknown (12-15).

The pharmacodynamics of the non-steroidal antiestrogenic compound tamoxifen has recently been reviewed in detail (16). The primary step is the competition with estradiol for binding to the estrogen receptor. At the chromatin level the mechanism of action is complex, and ultimately it leads to both partial block of the cell cycle in the early G_1-phase and to an increase in the concentration of the progesterone receptor protein in the tumor cells. Furthermore, recent studies have shown that tamoxifen binds to high-affinity, saturable sites that appear to be different from the estrogen receptor binding sites.

ABLATIVE THERAPY

The response rate after oophorectomy of premenopausal patients with advanced disease is approximately 30% (17), but with appreciable variation between the different samples, presumably owing to differences in selection criteria and in the definitions of response that were used (Table 2).

The median duration of response is about ten months. Similar response rates are achieved with both adrenalectomy and hypophysectomy (18).

Only a few randomized studies have been conducted to compare different ablative treatments. These include two trials with hypophysectomy versus adrenalectomy and oophorectomy (19,20) that yielded divergent results. In the first study, which included 144 patients, a higher response rate (36%) was found after hypophysectomy than after the combined treatment, whereas in the latter trial, which included 78 patients, similar rates were found in the two groups (22% versus 24%).

ADDITIVE THERAPY

As for ablative therapy, a wide range of response rates have been reported (Table 2) for both estrogen (15-38%) (17), androgen (10-38%) (17), and for progestins (9-54%) (15). Apart from various patient selection and response criteria, the different dose levels used in the individual trials may also account for some of the discrepancies. Thus, for estrogens the response rate seems to increase with an increasing daily dose from 1.5 mg and up to 1500 mg (21), and for androgens one (22) of two randomized trials (22,23) indicated a dose-response relationship. As concerns progestins, most of the earlier trials used daily doses of less than 0.5 g, but recent trials appear to demonstrate that the response rate rises when doses of 1-1.5 mg per day are used (15). However, the preliminary results of randomized trials have failed to demonstrate significantly different time to progression or survival with the two different dose levels (24,25), but more data on this subject are needed. Progestins have been

Table 2. Endocrine treatment in advanced breast cancer.

Reference	Treatment	Number of patients	Response rate	Range of response
17	Oophorectomy	1674	33 %	21 - 41 %
18	Adrenalectomy	4935	32 %	23 - 58 %
18	Hypophysectomy	1890	36 %	24 - 47 %
17	Estrogen	1683	26 %	15 - 38 %
17	Androgen	2250	21 %	10 - 38 %
15	Progesteron	783	31 %	9 - 54 %
26	Tamoxifen	1269	32 %	16 - 52 %
6	Aminoglute-thimide	909	32 %	25 - 50 %

administered both orally and intramuscularly but, so far, randomized trials analyzing the relation between the therapeutic efficacy and route of administration have not been published.

COMPETITIVE THERAPY

The average response rate with tamoxifen is 32% (Table 2), with a range form 16 to 52% (26). The most frequently used daily doses are 20-40 mg and randomized trials have demonstrated no significant differences in treatment results when comparing 30 mg with 90 mg daily (27) or 20 mg with 40 mg daily (28,29).

Recent years have seen a number of phase II studies with tamoxifen in premenopausal patients with advanced disease (30-34). The response is close to 30% and seems thus similar to that achieved with oophorectomy which was also confirmed in a small randomized comparison of oophorectomy and tamoxifen (35). However, additional data from randomized trials are needed.

INHIBITIVE THERAPY

The average response to treatment with aminoglutethimide supplemented by substitution with glucocorticoids is 31% (Table 2) with a range from 16 to 43% (6). Most studies have used a dose of aminoglutethimide of 1000 mg per day supplemented by hydrocortisone. A recent study demonstrated 500 mg and 1000 mg per day to be equally effective (36). More studies should be undertaken to analyse the role, with respect to response, of hydrocortisone.

Up to the present day only very preliminary data have been published for trilostane (37) and danazol (38).

LH-RH analogues are for the present being treated in phase II trials in premenopausal patients, but conclusive data are not yet available. However, preliminarily the efficacy seems to be similar to that achieved with oophorectomy.

TRIALS OF DIFFERENT THERAPIES

Table 3 reviews a number of randomized studies comparing competitive therapy to other forms of endocrine therapy.

Similar response rates were reported for tamoxifen and estrogen, but the side effects were significantly more pronounced in the group treated with estrogen (39-41).

In the comparative trial of tamoxifen versus androgen a lower response rate and more pronounced side effects were observed in patients treated with androgen (42).

Tamoxifen was compared with a progestin in 4 trials. The response rates were similar but the duration of response was longer and side effects less pronounced in the groups treated with tamoxifen (43-46).

More or less the same therapeutic results were obtained in the two trials in which tamoxifen was compared with aminoglutethimide, but side effects were more pronounced with the latter treatment (47,48).

TRIALS OF COMBINED THERAPIES

The comparable response rates achieved with the different endocrine therapies do not necessarily mean that the various treatments have the same ultimate mode of action and the considerable degree of cross-sensitivity and the lack of complete cross-resistance (49) suggest that combined methods of endocrine therapy might increase the therapeutic response.

In recent years a number of randomized trials have been published in which tamoxifen alone was been assessed against tamoxifen combined with other endorcine therapy. The results of some of these trials have recently been reviewed (50) and are briefly summarized in Table 4.

No difference was observed when estrogen was added to tamoxifen (51). When comparing tamoxifen to tamoxifen and the androgen fluoxymesterone, a significant difference in response rates, 15%

Table 3.

Randomized trials comparing tamoxifen to other endocrine therapies.

Reference	Treatment	Number of patients	Response rate
39 - 41	Tamoxifen	127	33 %
	Estrogens	130	35 %
42	Tamoxifen	37	30 %
	Androgens	42	19 %
46	Tamoxifen	140	30 %
	Progestins	141	27 %
47,48	Tamoxifen	99	33 %
	Aminoglute-thimide plus Hydrocortisone	93	32 %

versus 37%, was observed (52). It may be argued, however, that this trial was not conducted as an orthodox phase III study. Thus different doses of tamoxifen were used, from 2 mg/m^2 to 100 mg/m^2 twice daily, so that the number of patients who were given the optimum dose of tamoxifen may have been modest. In Heinonen's trial too (53), the response rate was higher after the combination therapy, but the difference was not significant. Tamoxifen combined with medroxyprogesterone acetate (MPA) produced lower response rates than tamoxifen alone (54), but the dose of MPA was rather low, 100 mg daily.

In one trial tamoxifen was compared to tamoxifen in combination with prednisolone. The combination treatment was significantly more effective than the single-drug therapy, for which the response rate was, in fact, remarkably low (55). However, in a subsequent similar comparison the preliminary data indicate the combination of tamoxifen and prednisolone to be superior to tamoxifen alone (56). In three trials no significant differences were observed between treatment with tamoxifen alone and tamoxifen in combination with aminoglutethimide (57-59), and in one small trial the addition of bromocriptin did not improve the efficacy (60). In the trial comparing tamoxifen with tamoxifen in combination with aminoglutethimide, hydrocortisone and danazol (61), the response rate was significantly superior with the combination; however, no differences in response durations or survivial times were observed.

Table 4.

Randomized trials comparing tamoxifen to tamoxifen in combination with other endocrine therapies.

Reference	Treatment	Number of patients	Response rate
51	TAM	65	39 %
	TAM+DES	57	37 %
52	TAM	52	15 %
	TAM+FLU	56	37 %
53	TAM	34	35 %
	TAM+NAND	44	43 %
54	TAM	46	44 %
	TAM+MPA	55	26 %
55	TAM	57	11 %
	TAM+PRED	61	33 %
57	TAM	26	19 %
	TAM+AG	26	23 %
58	TAM	96	26 %
	TAM+AG+H	75	39 %
59	TAM	27	34 %
	TAM+AG+H	28	28 %
60	TAM	23	22 %
	TAM+Br	20	20 %
61	TAM	99	31 %
	TAM+AG+H+D	99	43 %

ALTERNATING THERAPY

Treatment with tamoxifen is known to increase the content of progesterone receptors in the tumor tissue. For this reason alternating therapy with tamoxifen and progestins has been suggested, but data from larger trials are not yet available. This approach should also be extended to analyse the importance of prolonged treatment-free intervals between the alternating therapies with different agents.

RECRUITMENT

Alternating or repetitive use of cytotoxic and endocrine therapy has been proposed (62,63) as an approach by which non-dividing cells should be recruited and thereby optimize the effect of the cytotoxic drugs. Preliminary data have been disappointing (64-66), but this approach, which is theoretically attractive, has to be further elucidated in phase III trials.

CHOICE OF ENDOCRINE THERAPY

The choice of endocrine therapy will depend upon a balance between efficacy on the one hand, and toxicity of the therapy in question on the other. For premenopausal patients it is nowadays accepted that oophorectomy should be performed when endocrine therapy is indicated. However, preliminary data indicate that tamoxifen may be equally effective.

For postmenopausal patients the choice lies between additive, competitive and inhibitive therapy. From the results of the comparative studies of tamoxifen versus other endocrine therapies, it may be concluded that tamoxifen should be used as the endocrine therapy of choice in postmenopausal patients, whilst the other forms of treatment may be used as second-line endocrine therapy, depending on the response to primary treatment. Thus, in patients who responded to the primary therapy, the probability of a later response to secondary endocrine therapy was 48%, whereas it was only 12% in those who failed to respond to the initial endocrine therapy (49).

With the possible exception of combined tamoxifen-prednisolone, combined endocrine therapy, so far, has not proved superior to single agent therapy with tamoxifen.

CONCLUSION

The efficacy of endocrine treatment of advanced breast cancer is well established. However, among unselected patients the response rate remains approximately 30-35% and during endocrine therapy all the patients will ultimately experience progression of the disease.

A better understanding of the biology of breast cancer, a more complete knowledge of the modes of action of the different treatments and of the mechanism of the development of endocrine resistance are prerequisites for futher improvement in the endocrine treatment of advanced breast cancer.

REFERENCES

1. Dao TL: Ablation therapy for hormone-dependent tumours. Ann Rev Med 1972 (23):1-18
2. Robin PE and Dalton GA: The role of major endocrine ablation.In: Stoll BA (ed) Breast cancer management - early and late. Chicago Year Book 1977: 147-156
3. Hayward J: Hormones and human breast cancer. Recent Results in Cancer Research vol 24 1970 Berlin, Heidelberg, New York: Springer Verlag

4. Dao TL: The value of adrenalectomy in patients with metastatic breast cancer. Surg Clin North Am 1978 (58):801-807
5. Hayward JL, Atkins HJB and Falconer MA: Clinical trials comparing transfrontal hypophysectmomy with adrenalectomy and with transethmoidal hypophysectomy. In: Joslin CAF, Gleave En (eds) The clinical management of advanced breast cancer. Cardiff: Alpha Omega Alpha 1970:50-53
6. Stuart-Harris RC and Smith IE: Amiñoglutethimide in the treatment of advanced breast cancer. Cancer Treat Rev 1984 (2):189-204
7. Semple CG, Thomson JA, Stark AN, McDonald M and Beatstoll GH: Trilostane and the normal hypothalamic-pituatory-adrenocorticol axis. Clin Endocrinol 1982 (17):569-575
8. Chamness GC, Asch RH and Paurstein CJ: Danazol binding and translocation of steroid receptors. Am J Obstet Gynecol 1980 (136):426-429
9. Menon M, Azhar S and Menon KMJ: Evidence that danazol inhibits gonadotropin-induced ovarian sterodogenesis at a point distal to gonadotropin receptor interaction and adonosine 3' 5' - cyclic monophosphate formation. Am J Obstet Gynecol 1980 (136):524-530
10. Jenkin G: The mechanism of action of danazol. A novel steroid derivative. Aust N Z J Obstet Gynecol 1980 (2):113-118
11. Furr BJA and Nicholson RI: Use of analogues of luteinizing hormone-releasing hormone for the treatment of cancer. J Reprod Fertil 1982 (64):529-539
12. Lippman M, Bolan G and Hoff K: The effects of estrogens and antiestrogens on hormone-responsive Human Breast Cancer in Long-Term Tissue Culture. Cancer Res 1976 (36):4595-4601
13. Zava DT and McGuire WL: Human breast cancer: Androgen action mediated by estrogen receptor. Science 1978 (199):787-788
14. Nicholson RJ, Davies P and Griffiths K: Interaction of androgens with oestradiol-lytic mechanism. Eur J Cancer 1978 (14):439-445
15. Lober J, Rose C, Salimtschik M and Mouridsen HTL: Treatment of advanced breast cancer with progestins. Acta Obstet Gynecol Scand (suppl.) 1981 (101):39-47
16. Furr BJA and Jordan VC: The pharmacoloy and clinical uses of tamoxifen. Pharma Ther 1984 (25):127-205
17. Henderson IC and Canellos GP: Cancer of the breast. The past decade (First of two parts). New Engl J Med 1980 (302):17-30
18. Robin PE and Dalton GA: The role of major endocrine ablation. In: Stoll BA (ed) Breast cancer management early and late. 1977: 147-153 London:Heineman
19. Hayward JL, Atkins and HJB Falconer MA: Clinical trials comparing transfrontal hypophysectomy with adrenalectomy and with transethmoidal hypophysectomy. In: Joslin CAF and Gleave EN (eds) The clinical management of advanced Breast Cancer. Cardiff: Alpha Omega Alpha 1970: 50-53
20. Roberts MM: A comparison of transethmoidal hypophysectomy, Yttrium 90 implant and adrenalectomy. In: Joslin CAF, Gleave EN (eds) The clinical management of advanced breast cancer Cardiff: Alpha Omega Alpha 1970: 54-62

21. Carter AC, Sedransk N and Kelley RM: Diethylstilbestrol: recommended dosages for different categories of breast cancer patients: Report of the Cooperative Breast Cancer Group. JAMA 1977 (237):2079-2085
22. Volk H, Deupree RH, Goldenberg IS, Wilden RC, Carabasi RA and Escher P: A dose response evaluation of delta-1-testolactone in advanced breast cancer. Cancer 1974 (9):33-39
23. Talley RW, Haines CR and Waters MN: A dose-response evaluation of androgens in the treatment of metastatic breast cancer. Cancer 1973 (32):315-320
24. Cavalli F, Goldhirsch A, Jungi WF, Martz G and ALbert P: Low- versus high-dose medroxyprogesterone acetate in the treatment of advanced breast cancer. Excerpta Medica International Congress Series 1982 (64):224
25. Kamby C, Engelsman E, Nooy M, Rose C, Mouridsen HT, Sylvester R and Rotmenz N: Treatment of advanced breast cancer with medroxyprogesterone acetate: A phase III trial. 2nd European conference on clinical oncology and cancer nursing. Amsterdam 1983 abstract No 17-29
26. Mouridsen HT, Palshof T, Patterson J and Batterby L: Tamoxifen in advanced breasr cancer. Cancer Treatm Rev 1978 (5):131-141
27. McGuire WL: Hormone receptors: their role in predicting prognosis and response to endocrine therapy. Semin Oncol 1978 (5):428
28. Ward HWC: Anti-oestrogen therapy for breast cancer: a trial of tamoxifen at two-dose levels. Br Med J 1973 (1):13-14
29. Bratherton DG, Brown CH, Buchanan R, Halle V, Kingsley Pillers EM, Wheeler TK and Williams CJ: A comparison of two doses of tamoxifen (Nolvadex) in postmenopausal women with advanced breast cancer: 10 mg b.d. vs 20 mg b.d. Br J Cancer 1984 (50):199-205
30. Hoogstraten B, Fletcher WS, Gad-el-Mowla N, Maloney T, Altman SJ, Vaughn CB and Faulker MA: Tamoxifen and oophorectomy in the treatment of recurrent breast cancer: A Southwest Oncology Group Study. Cancer Res 1982 (42):4788-4791
31. Manni A and Pearson OH: Antiestrogen-induced remissions in premenopausal women with stage IV breast cancer: effects on ovarian function. Cancer Treatm 1980 (64):779-785
32. Pritchard KI, Thomson DB, Myers RE, Sutherland DJD, Mobbs BG and Meakin JW: Tamoxifen therapy in premenopausal patients with metastatic breast cancer. Cancer Treatm Rep 1980 (64):787-796
33. Planting AST, Alexieva-Figusch J, Blonk-vd Wijst J and van Putten WLJ: Tamoxifen therapy in premenopausal women with metastatic breast cancer. Cancer Treatm Rep 1985 : 363-368
34. Wada T, Koyama H and Teresawa T: Effect of tamoxifen in premenopausal Japanese women with advanced breast cancer. Cancer Treatment Rep 1981 (65):728-729
35. Ingle JN, Krook JE, Gree SJ, Kubista TP, Evanson LL, Almann DL, Chang MN, Bisel HF, Windschitl HE, TWito SI and Pfeifle DM: Randomized trial of bilateral oophorectomy versus tamoxifen in premenopausal women with metastatic breast cancer. J Clin Oncol 1986 (4):178-185
36. Bonneterre J, Coppens H, Mauriac L, Metz M, Rouesse J, Armand JP, Fargeot P, Mathieu M, Tubiana M and Cappelaere

P: Aminoglutethimide in advanced breast cancer: Clinical results of a French multicenter randomized trial comparing 500 mg and 1 g/day. Eur J Cancer Clin Oncol 1985 (21):1153-1158

37. Hindley AC: Trilostane. A new hormonal agent in breast cancer. 3rd EORTC Breast Cancer Working Conf. Abstract no IX, 21, 1983

38. Coombs RC, Dearnaley D, Humphreys J, Gazet JC, Ford HT, Bash AG, Mashiter K and Powles TJ: Danazol treatment for advanced breast cancer. Eur J Cancer (suppl) 1980 (1):83-88

39. Stewart HJ, Forrest APM and Gunn JM: The tamoxifen trial-a double-blind comparison with stilbestrol in postmenopausal women with advanced breast cancer. Eur J Cancer (suppl) 1980 (1):83-88

40. Beex L, Pieters G, Smals A, Koenders A, Benraad T and Kloppenberg P: Tamoxifen vs ethinyl estradiol in the treatment of postmenopausal women with advanced breast cancer. Cancer Treat Rep 1981 (65):179-185

41. Ingle JN, Ahmann DL, Green SJ, Edmonson JH, Bisel JH, Kvals LK, Nichols WC, Creagan ET, Hahn RG, Rubin J and Frytag S: Randomized clinical trial of diethylstilbestrol vs tamoxifen in postmenopausal women with advanced breast cancer. N Engl J Med 1980 (304):16-21

42. Westerberg H: Tamoxifen and fluoxymesterone in advanced breast cancer: a controlled clinical trial. Cancer Treat Rep 1980 (64):117-121

43. Ingle JN, Creagan ET, Ahmann DL, Hahn RG, Green SJ, Rubin J and Edmonson JH: Randomized clinical trial of megestrol acetate versus tamoxifen in paramenopausal or castrated women with advanced breast cancer. Am J Clin Oncol 1982 (5):155-160

44. Morgan LR and Donley PJ: Tamoxifen versus megestrol acetate in breast cancer. Rev Endocr Rel Cancer (Suppl) 1981 (9):301-310

45. Beretta G, Tabiadon D, Tedeschi L and Luporini G: Hormone therapy of advanced breast carcinoma: Comparative evaluation of tamoxifen citrate versus medroxyprogesterone acetate, In: Iacobelli S (ed) Role of Tamoxifen in Breast Cancer New York: Raven Press 1982: 113-120

46. Pannuti F, Martoni A, Fruet F, Burroni P, Canova N and Hall S: Oral high dose medroxyprogesterone acetate versus tamoxifen in postmenopausal patients with advanced breast cancer. In: Iacobelli S (ed) The role of Tamoxifen in Breast Cancer. New York: Raven Press 1982: 85-92

47. Liptoarvey HA, Santen RJ, Boucher A, White D, Bernath A, Dixon R, Richards G and Shafik A: Randomized trial of aminoglutethimide versus tamoxifen in metastatic breast cancer. Cancer Res (suppl) 1982 (42):3434-3436

48. Smith IE, HArris AL, Morgan M, Gazet JC and McKinna SA: Tamoxifen versus aminoglutethimide versus combined tamoxifen and aminoglutethimide in the treatment of advanced breast carcinoma. Cancer Res (suppl 42) 1982: 3430-3433

49. Rose C and Mouridsen HT: Combined cytotoxic and endocrine therapy in advanced breast cancer. In: Bresciani F, King RBJ, Lippman ME, Namer M, Raynud JP (eds) Progress in cancer research and therapy. New York: Raven Press 1984: 269-286

50. Rose C and Mouridsen HT: Treatment of advanced breast cancer with tamoxifen. Recent Results Cancer Res. 1984 (91):230-242

51. Mouridsen HT, Salimtschik M, Dombernowsky P, Gelshoj K, Palshof T, Rorth M, Daehnfeldt JL and Rose C: Therapeutic effect of tamoxifen versus combined tamoxifen and diethylstibestrol in advanced breast cancer in post-menopausal women. Eur J Cancer (suppl) 1980 (1):107-110

52. Tormey DC, Lippman MF, Edwards BE and Cassedy J: Evaluation of tamoxifen doses with and without fluoxymestrone in advanced breast cancer. Ann Intern Med 1983 (98):139-144

53. Heinonen E, Alanko A, Grohn P and Rissanen P: Tamoxifen versus nandrolone-decanoate in advanced breast cancer. 1st Scand Breast Cancer Sypmposium, Aarhus, Denmark 1982 Abstract 28

54. Mouridsen HT, Ellemann K, Mattson W, Palshof T: Therapeutic effect of tamoxifen versus tamoxifen combined with medroxyprogesterone acetate in advanced breast cancer in postmenopausal women. Cancer Treat Rep 1979 (63):171-175

55. Stewart JF, Rubens RD, King RJB, Minton MJ, Steiner R, Tong D, Winter PJ, Knoght RK and Hayward JL: Contribution of prednisolone to the primary endocrine treatment of advanced breast cancer. Eur J Canc Clin Oncol 1982 (18):1307-1314

56. Rubens RD and Knight RK: The contribution of prednisolone (P) to primary endocrine therapy (PET) in advanced breast cancer. ASCO C 202, 1985

57. Milsted E, Habeshow T, Sangster G, Kaye S and Calman K: Tamoxifen versus tamoxifen with aminoglutethimide in postmenopausal women with advanced breast cancer. 2nd Eur Conference on Clinical Oncology and Cancer Nursing. Amsterdam 1983. Abstract p. 186

58. Ingle JN, Green SJ, Ahmann Dl, Edmonson JH, Nichols WC, Frytag S and Rubin J: Progress report on two clinical trials in women with advanced breast cancer. Trial I: Tamoxifen versus tamoxifen plus aminoglutethimide; Trial II: Aminoglutethimide in patients with prior tamoxifen exposuncer Res (suppl) 1982 (42):3461-3467

59. Rose C, Kamby C, Mouridsen HT, Bastholt L, Brincker H, Skovgaard-Poulsen H, Andersen AP, Loft H, Dombernowsky P and Andersen KW: Combined endocrine treatment of postmenopausal patients with advanced breast cancer. A randomized trial of tamoxifen vs tamoxifen plus aminoglutethimide and hydrocortisone. Breast Cancer Res and Treatm 1986. In press

60. Settatree RS: Bromocriptine, prolactine and nolvadex in advanced breast cancer. Revs Endocr Rel Cancer (suppl) 1980 (5):63-70

61. Powles TJ, Ashley S and Ford HT: Treatment of disseminated breast cancer with tamoxifen, aminoglutethimide, hydrocortisone and danazol used in combination or sequentially. Lancet 1984 (1):1369-1373

62. Lippman ME: Efforts to comibine endocrine and chemotherapy in the management of breast cancer: Do two and two equal three? Breast Cancer Res and Treatm 1983 (3):117-127

63. Osborne CK: Combined chemo-endocrine therapy in breast

cancer: A hypothesis. Breast Cancer Res and Treatm 1981 (1):121-123

64. Lippman ME, Cassidy J, Wesley M and Young RC: A randomized attempt to increase the efficacy of cytotoxic chemotherapy in metastatic breast cancer by hormonal synchronization. J Clin Oncol 1984 (2):28-35

65. Allegra JC: Methotrexate and 5-fluorouracil following tamoxifen and premarin in advanced breast cancer. Semin Oncol (suppl) 1983 (2):23-28

66. Paridaens R, Blonk van der Wijst J, Juline JP, Ferrazzi E, Claysse A, Heuson JC, Sylvester R and Rotmenz N: Cyclic combination chemotherapy preceded by estrogenic recruitment for treatment of advanced breast cancer. A phase II trial of the EORTC Breast Cancer Cooperative Group. 3rd EORTC Breast Cancer Working Conference 1983. Abstract n. 1, 10

Endocrine Aspects in Adjuvant Therapy for Early Breast Cancer

A. Goldhirsch*, R. D. Gelber**, and H. Mouridsen***

*Ludwig Institute for Cancer Research (Bern Branch), Inselspital, Bern, Switzerland
**Harvard School of Public Health and Dana-Farber Cancer Institute, Boston, MA, USA
***Finsen Institute, Copenhagen, Denmark

Despite controversy, adjuvant treatment (chemo- and/or hormone therapy) has become widely used in the management of breast cancer as an accepted means of improving disease-free survival and reducing mortality due to the disease (1,2). Two observations have been made during the past century:

1. Most of the patients with breast cancer relapse and die due to the disease, mainly because of development of distant metastases which, though occult, are established by the time the disease is diagnosed.

2. A substantial proportion of the patients with advanced breast cancer will have a regression of disease if hormonal treatments such as oophorectomy or administration of various hormonal agents are applied. However, metastatic disease has proven to be incurable with available means.

As a consequence of these observations, the next development in the treatment of breast cancer was the application of a systemic therapy during a period of time before metastases were clinically detectable in an attempt to eradicate microfoci of tumor cells and thereby achieve cure in a proportion of patients. Studies in animal models in fact demonstrated that, during the preclinical phase of metastatic disease, tumor cells are more vulnerable and can be eliminated.

The first clinical studies investigating the possibility of curing a proportion of patients via endocrine manipulation were initiated almost 40 years ago. The first of these concerned the use of either surgical oophorectomy or ovarian irradiation immediately after mastectomy as a means of endocrine manipulation. In the 1970s it was demonstrated that for postmenopausal patients with advanced disease, tamoxifen was an active agent (3). The use of tamoxifen in the adjuvant setting has been the subject of many trials in Europe and the United States. The purpose of this report is to discuss the endocrine aspects of adjuvant systemic therapy and to formulate hypotheses upon which future clinical investigations may be based. Some specific designs for future randomized clinical trials will be suggested. The first generation (1978-1981) of the Ludwig Breast Cancer Study Group trials was dedicated to the investigation of the endocrine components of adjuvant treatment in early breast cancer. The evidence from these trials will form the basis for a summary review of the literature.

Table 1. Randomized Trials with Adjuvant Oophorectomy (Ox) (either surgically or radiation induced)

Trial	(Ref)	No.Pts.	Yrs follow-up	Findings (remarks in parentheses)
Christie	(4)	598	15	Survival advantage for Ox: at 10 yrs 55% vs 48% at 15 yrs 45% vs 40%
Toronto	(5)	308	15	Survival advantage for Ox + low-dose continuous prednisone (p) in women 45 yrs old or older (72% vs 44%)
Saskatchewan	(6)	359	10	Survival advantage for Ox at 10 yrs (11% difference)
Ludwig II	(7)	327	5	No effect of additional Ox to combination chemotherapy with CMFp

A. Premenopausal women with early breast cancer

Some of the studies related to the effect of adjuvant oophorectomy are summarized in Table 1. The Christie, the Toronto and the Saskatchewan trials included mastectomy-alone treatment arms as a control. The results of the oldest of these were to some extent known when, in 1978, the Ludwig Breast Cancer Study Group launched their Trial II. Still other trials had shown that for premenopausal patients with metastases in one to three axillary nodes, chemotherapy, and especially the cyclophosphamide, methotrexate and 5-fluorouracil (CMF) combination, yielded significant benefit in terms of disease-free survival (DFS) and overall survival (OS) (8). This appeared to be less effective in premenopausal women with four or more axillary nodes involved.

In Ludwig II, 356 premenopausal and perimenopausal patients with metastases in four or more axillary lymph nodes were randomly allocated to receive either CMF with low-dose continuous prednisone (p), or surgical oophorectomy (Ox) followed by CMFp (Figure 1).

The aim of the trial was to evaluate the impact of adding ovarian ablation to combination chemotherapy. At a median follow-up of five years, the outcome (Kaplan-Meier five-year percentage plus/minus standard error) by assigned treatment group was similar for DFS (CMFp = 43% ± 4% vs Ox + CMFp = 48% ± 4%) and for overall survival (61% ± 4% vs 65% ± 4%, respectively). Adhering to the principle of intent to treat eligible patients, the analyses were carried out on the entire population (eligible = 327 patients). The conclusions as to the treatment effectiveness, however, did not change in analyses that excluded 22 patients who did not receive the assigned treatment.

Figure 1. LUDWIG BREAST CANCER STUDIES (FIRST GENERATION) Patients Entered from July 1978 to August 1981

Study		Patients		Treatment	No evaluable
Ludwig I	SURGERY	PRE-MENOPAUSAL 1 - 3 N+	RANDOM	CMF	241
				CMFp	250
Ludwig II	SURGERY	PRE-MENOPAUSAL 4 or more N+	RANDOM	CMFp	161
				oophorectomy +CMFp	166
Ludwig III	SURGERY	POST-MENOPAUSAL ALL N+ 65 years old or less	RANDOM	Observation	156
				CMFp + T	154
				p + T	153
Ludwig IV	SURGERY	POST-MENOPAUSAL All N+ 66 to 80 years old	RANDOM	Observation	153
				p + T	167

Treatment:
C: cyclophosphamide 100 mg/m^2 orally days 1 - 14
M: methotrexate 40 mg/m^2 i.v. days 1 and 8
F: 5-fluorouracil 600 mg/m^2 i.v. days 1 and 8
CMF: q 28 days for 12 cycles
p: prednisone 7.5 mg/day orally (5 mg a.m.; 2.5 mg p.m.)
T: tamoxifen 10 mg b.i.d. orally
p and T continuously for 12 months

Oophorectomy is guaranteed to provide complete loss of ovarian function. Chemotherapy, especially with the alkylating agents which are included in the CMF combination, is known to cause amenorrhea due to suppression of gonadal activity. The amenorrhea observed in this trial for patients receiving only CMFp (89% of them) may have reflected a loss of endocrine ovarian function having an impact similar to that of oophorectomy. Thus the addition of surgical oophorectomy to the adjuvant chemotherapy regimen may have been rendered superfluous by this effect of cytotoxic treatment. Furthermore, continuous administration of low-dose prednisone in both treatment regimens might exert an additional antineoplastic effect via endocrine mechanisms (i.e., suppression of adrenal function).

Retrospective analyses of subgroup populations revealed the unexpected difference in favor of oophorectomy + CMFp in the patients with PR-negative tumors (Figure 2.)

Because of the possibility that multiple subgroup analyses produce spurious differences in treatment outcome, caution must be observed in the interpretation of this result within a subgroup. The combination of chemo- and endocrine therapy may, however, be more effective in patients with tumors containing few or no receptors, as suggested by the results from other trials (Ludwig III and ECOG) (9,10,11). A review of the studies involving oophorectomy (Table 1), and the observation that as yet no advantage has been perceived by the addition of oophorectomy to a combination chemotherapy (CMFp in the Ludwig II), may lead to the hypothesis that oophorectomy at best yields results similar to those of adjuvant chemotherapy. A direct comparison to test this hypothesis in a prospective study has not yet been performed.

A further question might be formulated as to whether adjuvant chemotherapy acts in premenopausal women as a chemical

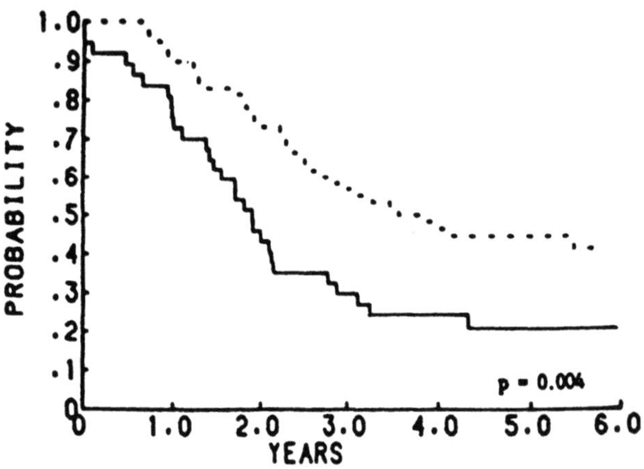

Treatment	FAIL	TOTAL	5-YEAR DFS RATE
—— CMFp	29	37	21%
··· CMFp + Ox	35	60	45%

Figure 2. Ludwig II - Disease-free survival - PR-negative

oophorectomy. The effect of chemotherapy may be mediated primarily through its effect on the endocrine system. Mechanisms might include both suppression of ovarian function and, in part, reduction of steroid hormone production in the adrenals. Data in support of this hypothesis might be derived from the Ludwig Trial I: 505 premenopausal and perimenopausal patients with metastases in 1-3 axillary lymph nodes were randomly allocated to receive either CMF or CMFp to evaluate the impact of adding low-dose prednisone to combination chemotherapy (Figure 1). The trial was extensively described in a recent publication (12). 491 patients were evaluable for analysis of outcome. The 5-year disease-free survival was similar in the two treatment groups (CMF = 71% ± 3% vs CMFp = 68% ± 3%) as well as overall survival rates (85% ± 2% vs 84% ± 2%, respectively). As previously described (12), patients in the CMFp-treated group received significantly higher doses of CMF than patients who did not receive prednisone. On the average, 72% of the full CMF dose in cycles 1-6 was received by CMF-treated patients compared with 83% of the CMFp-treated patients. This was mainly due to less hematological toxicity experienced by the CMFp-treated patients. 399 patients were evaluable for a subgroup analysis of disease-free survival by induced amenorrhea (Figure 3).

A multivariate analysis of treatment effects and known prognostic variables revealed that the impact on disease-free survival of amenorrhea, age (40 years or more vs 39 years or less), estrogen receptor content in the primary (ER+ vs ER-), and the average dose of CMF delivered were all confounded. In fact, the positive effect of amenorrhea on prognosis (DFS) was seen only in the younger group of patients, in patients with ER-positive tumors and, an interesting observation, in patients who had received an average CMF dose of 80% or less. In patients who received more than 80% of the average CMF dose the outcome was similar whether they developed amenorrhea or not. Similar retrospective analyses of outcome by amenorrhea have been conducted for other trials (Table 2).

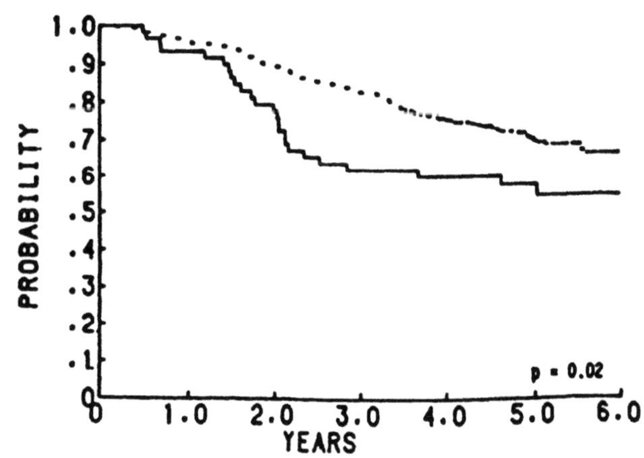

Amenorrhea	NED	FAIL	TOTAL	5-YEAR DFS RATES
—— No	34	25	59	58%
··· Yes	240	100	340	70%

Figure 3. Ludwig I - Disease-free survival

Table 2 Reported Amenorrhea in Randomized Trials Using Adjuvant Chemotherapy in Premenopausal Patients

Trial	(Ref)	No Pts evaluable	Treatment	Findings
Ludwig I	(12)	491	CMF CMFp	Amenorrhea (A) associated with DFS and OS Advantage (see text). At 5 years DFS 70% for A vs 58% for non-A (p=0.02)
Danish Group	(13)	1029	C CMF Control	DFS advantage for pts with A vs non-A in the C-treated group but not in the CMF group
Milan	(14)	386	CMF Control	Non-statistically-significant difference for DFS of pts with CMF-induced A (4-year rates 73% vs 56%)
NSABP	(15)	349	L-PAM Control	No difference between pts with and without A
ECOG	(16)	369	CMF CMFP CMFP+T	Survival advantage for pts with A
Guy's/Christie	(17)	407	CMF Control	DFS advantage for pts with A (CMF dose about 20% less than in Milan study)

The fact that amenorrhea seems to be associated with a better outcome in the majority of the studies validates the hypothesis that at least some of the effectiveness of the cytotoxic combination in premenopausal women is due to suppression of ovarian endocrine activity. However, because induced amenorrhea does not improve DFS among patients who receive full doses of chemotherapy, some direct cytotoxic activity must be postulated. The extent to which the chemotherapy effect is mediated via endocrine mechanisms should, however, be prospectively investigated.

What are the questions to be asked by trials conducted for clarification of the role of endocrine mechanisms in delaying recurrence and reducing deaths in premenopausal patients? Table 3 describes hypothetical trial designs relevant to endocrine mechanisms in adjuvant settings.

Table 3 Hypothetical designs to investigate endocrine mechanisms in adjuvant setting in premenopausal patients

---

A. Induced amenorrhea

Population of interest: premenopausal patients with steroid hormone receptor positive tumors

CT x

6 months : if amenorrhea, observe

if no amenorrhea : randomize
- oophorectomy
- observation

B. Induced suppression of ovarian or adrenal function with pharmacological means (endocrine therapy) (with same population of interest as A.)

Randomize
- CT
- (CT + Endocrine therapy)
- Endocrine therapy alone

C. Combined chemo-endocrine therapy in premenopausal patients with tumors which contain low concentrations of or no hormone receptors

Randomize
- CT
- CT + Endocrine therapy

A and B include investigations in patients with steroid receptor hormone-containing tumors, while C relates to an investigation in premenopausal patients with tumors which contain low or no hormone receptors. The design in this case is motivated by the necessity to verify the unexpected results of the retrospective analysis of Ludwig Trial II (patients with PgR-negative tumors).

Other findings of treatment interaction effects within patient subgroups deserve further study. Adding tamoxifen to combination chemotherapy reduced DFS and overall survival for younger patients (less than 50 years old) whose tumors contained low or no progesterone receptors in the NSABP B-09 protocol (18). These data have been interpreted as indicating that tamoxifen therapy is detrimental for this subgroup of patients. Treatment effect interactions as well as the characteristics of the subpopulation might be responsible for the observed poor result. Patients in the B-09 study all received a specific chemotherapy regimen (L-pam + 5-fluorouracil administered once every 6 weeks) with or without tamoxifen. This chemotherapy differs substantially from the CMF types of regimens used by other groups. It might be hypothesized that a more frequent administration of effective cytotoxic drugs increases kill of cells that escape the growth

Table 4 Some Randomized Trials with Adjuvant Tamoxifen in Postmenopausal Patients

Trial	(Ref)	No evaluable pts	Treatment duration	Findings (remarks in parentheses)
Copenhagen	(19)	94	2 years	DFS advantage for treated patients
Danish	(20)	1647	1 year	DFS advantage for treated patients (postoperative radiotherapy). No survival difference
Swedish	(21)	865	2 years	DFS advantage for treated patients (postoperative RT to high-risk population)
Christie	(22)	588	1 year	No survival difference for treated patients
NATO	(23)	1124 pre- + postmen.	2 years	DFS and OS advantage for treated patients
Toronto	(24)	366	2 years	DFS advantage for treated patients (only the series without postoperative radiotherapy)
ECOG	(23)	170	2 years	DFS advantage for treated patients
Ludwig III+IV	(26)	629	1 year	DFS advantage for treated patients (low-dose prednisone given with tamoxifen) (see test)

arrest caused by tamoxifen therapy. This could explain why other groups do not find the same substantial negative effects of combined tamoxifen and chemotherapy in the premenopausal, PgR-negative subgroup. Strong treatment-related and host-feature-related interaction effects are quite likely to exist for hormone-dependent tumors. Especially, because the precise pathways of action of the variety of treatment applied are not completely understood, careful consideration of the details of patient selection and therapies administered must be given to the proper interpretation of trial results.

B. Postmenopausal patients

The DFS advantage of adjuvant chemotherapy compared with no adjuvant treatment was less for postmenopausal women than for premenopausal patients. The anti-estrogen tamoxifen, which was found to be a non-toxic and effective therapy for advanced breast cancer (3), was adopted for adjuvant use in trials which began simultaneously in the late 1970s throughout the world. Some of the randomized trials using tamoxifen and having a surgery-alone control group are described in Table 4. In overviews of trials recently conducted, the use of tamoxifen has been shown to reduce the mortality of breast cancer, especially for patients of 50 years of age or older.

In order to highlight the issues concerning endocrine adjuvant therapy in postmenopausal patients, the Ludwig Trials III and IV will be described.

In 1978 the Ludwig Breast Cancer Study Group initiated two trials in postmenopausal patients, both comparing the endocrine therapy with tamoxifen and prednisone to a surgery alone control group (Figure 1). A combined stratified analysis of 629 evaluable postmenopausal patients with axillary nodal metastases who received either p+T or no adjuvant therapy has been conducted at 60 months of median observation time. The 5-year results by treatment for all evaluable patients and for the subgroups defined according to estrogen receptor status are described in Table 5.

Patients with ER-positive tumors benefited from p+T in terms of disease-free survival. No benefit was observed for the endocrine treatment in the subpopulation with ER-negative tumors. Among the patients with ER-positive tumors the disease-free survival advantage for endocrine therapy was greater for those 65 years old or less (Ludwig III: 54% $\pm$ 8% vs 33% $\pm$ 7%, p=0.02) than for those 66 years old or more (Ludwig IV: 46% $\pm$ 7% vs 45% $\pm$ 8%, p=0.35).

The analysis of sites of first failure indicated a reduction in local, regional and contralateral breast cancer recurrence but not of distant metastases in the p+T-treated group (Table 6).

In a similar analysis restricted to the patients with known estrogen receptor status the reduction of these recurrences was seen exclusively within the group of patients with ER-positive tumors. It is hypothesized that the effect of endocrine adjuvant therapy with p+T is confined to those patients with ER-positive tumors and that the effect is quantitatively (but not qualitatively) greater in the young postmenopausal population (age 65 years or less). These results are similar to those observed by the Danish group (20).

Table 5 Ludwig III + IV : Combined analyses (p+T vs observation)
5-year DFS and OS Rates at 60 Months' Median Follow-up
(Kaplan-Meier % ± S.E.)

All Patients	No	DFS	OS
Observation	(309)	34 ± 3*	61 ± 3
p+T	(320)	43 ± 3*	63 ± 3
ER+			
Observation	(100)	39 ± 5*	73 ± 5
p+T	(104)	50 ± 5	73 ± 5
ER-			
Observation	(50)	30 ± 7	46 ± 7
p+T	(51)	25 ± 6	38 ± 7

* statistically significant differences; 2-sided logrank p<0.05

Table 6 Sites of First Failure Ludwig III and IV
60 Months Median Follow-up
(No. of deaths in parentheses)

	Observation		p ± T	
Scar alone	49 (17)		28 (12)	
Contralateral breast alone	8 (1)		1 (0)	
Loc/Reg without distant	45 (27)		22 (19)	
Distant	97 (66)		102 (71)	
Soft tissue		4 (2)		2 (1)
Bone		42 (24)		50 (31)
Viscera		51 (40)		50 (39)
Second primary (not breast)	5 (4)		6 (4)	
Death w/o recurrence	10 (10)		20 (20)	
Total Failed	214 (125)		179 (126)	
Total Cases	309		320	

Table 7 Randomized Trials with Adjuvant Combined Chemotherapy and Tamoxifen in Postmenopausal Patients

Trial	(Ref)	No evaluable pts	Treatments	Findings
NASBP	(18)	1861 pre- + postmen.	PF PFT	Advantage in DFS and OS for postmen pts with progesterone receptors ≥10 fmol (6-year results)
Case Western	(27)	312 pre- + postmen.	CMF CMF + T ± BCG	Advantage in DFS for pts with ER+ tumors (44-month results)
ECOG	(16)	369 premen.	CMF CMFP CMFP+T	No difference in outcome (4-year results)
ECOG	(11)	224 postmen.	CMFP CMFP+T Control	Advantage in DFS for CMFP+T in ER- subpopulation (4-year results)
Ludwig III	(9)	463 postmen.	CMFp+T p+T control	Advantage in DFS for CMFp+T vs P+T and vs control. Emerging OS advantage CMFp+T vs control (5-year results). Subgroup analysis (see text)

Whether chemotherapy alone might yield better results than tamoxifen alone in postmenopausal patients is not yet known. An ongoing trial by the Southwest Oncology Group (SWOG) is addressing this question for patients with ER-positive tumors. The combination of chemo-endocrine therapy has, however, been extensively investigated during the past decade. Some of the trials addressing this question are described in Table 7.

Table 8: Ludwig III : 5-year DFS and Overall Survival (OS) Rates at 60 Months of Median Follow-up (Kaplan-Meier % ± S.E.)

All Patients	(No.)	DFS		OS
Observation	(156)	31 ± 4*		59 ± 4**
p+T	(153)	41 ± 4*		64 ± 4
CMFp+T	(154)	59 ± 4*		71 ± 4**
ER+				
Observation	(53)	33 ± 7	*	72 ± 6
p+T	(45)	54 ± 8		82 ± 6
CMFp+T	(58)	59 ± 7		76 ± 6
ER-				
Observation	(33)	28 ± 8		47 ± 9
p+T	(30)	23 ± 8	*	39 ± 9
CMFp+T	(19)	63 ± 11		63 ± 11

* statistically significant differences; 2-sided logrank p-value = 0.05

** 2-sided logrank p-value = 0.07

The corresponding trial from the first generation of the Ludwig studies is Trial III (Figure 1). 503 patients were randomized to one of the three treatment options and 463 postmenopausal patients 65 years old or younger were evaluable. The 5-year results by treatment for all evaluable patients and for the subgroups defined according to estrogen receptor status are described in Table 8 and in Figures 4 and 5.

For patients with ER-positive tumors the DFS of the CMFp+T group and of the p+T group were similar. For those with ER-negative tumors the DFS was significantly longer for the CMFp+T treated patients than for both the p+T group and the observation group. Interestingly, in their account of the results from the ECOG trial, Taylor et al (11) also report an advantage for CMFp+T compared with either CMFp or control in the subpopulation with

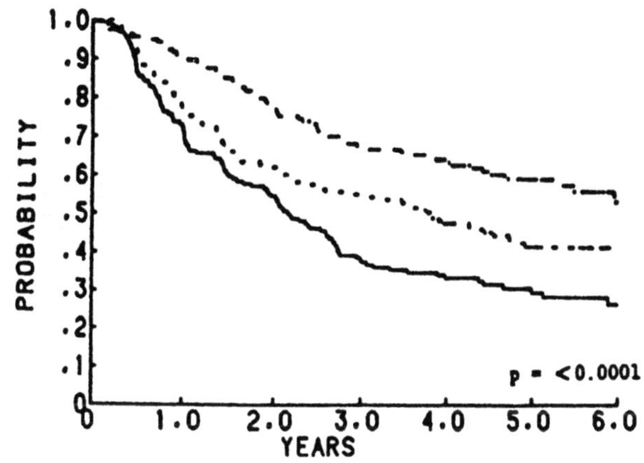

Treatment	FAIL	TOTAL	5-YEAR DFS RATE
—— Obs	110	156	31%
··· p + T	87	153	41%
- - CMFp + T	64	154	59%

Figure 4. Ludwig II - Disease-free survival

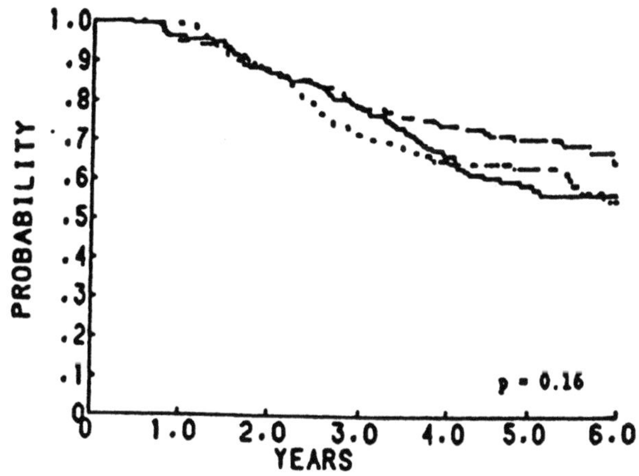

Treatment	DEAD	TOTAL	5-YEAR OS RATE
—— Obs	65	156	59%
··· p + T	61	153	64%
- - CMFp + T	47	154	71%

Figure 5. Overall survival

ER-negative tumors. This retrospective analysis provides the basis for the hypothesis that a CMFp combination plus tamoxifen might improve the results of patients whose tumors contain low or no steroid hormone receptors.

Examples of hypothetical trial designs for investigating endocrine therapy in postmenopausal patients are listed in Table 9.

The effect of combined chemo-endocrine therapy in relation to known receptor status should be investigated prospectively (Table 9). The sample size considerations should be made separately for each subpopulation. Testing the effects of combined endocrine agents in patients with hormone receptor-containing tumors vs a single agent would be of interest. The combination of prednisone and tamoxifen has repeatedly been shown to be superior in advanced disease in terms of remission rate and of overall survival (28). The randomized comparison in the adjuvant setting is therefore important. Studies are also needed to analyse the importance of duration of adjuvant tamoxifen and the effect of

Table 9 Hypothetical trial designs to investigate endocrine therapies in postmenopausal patients

A. The effect of combined chemo-endocrine therapy by known receptor status

ER+ *

Randomize → CT + Tamoxifen / Tamoxifen

ER- *

* Similar trial for the two subpopulations

B. The effect of a combination endocrine therapy in patients with ER+ tumors

Randomize → Tamoxifen + prednisone / Tamoxifen

C. The effect of sequential hormonal therapies in patients with ER+ tumors

Randomize → Agent A→, agent B upon relapse / Agent A for established time, then switch to B sequential hormonal therapies, especially those which exert cytotoxicity in a different way (e.g., antiestrogens, aromarase inhibitors, LHRH analogs etc.).

It is important to note that a trial in patients with operable breast cancer is an exercise which bears fruit only some years after formulation of the hypotheses which led to its conception and conduct. The results of a trial almost always lead to the formulation of new hypotheses which the trial itself fails to confirm. Because of the biology of breast cancer (a low and constant yearly relapse rate), and of the expected limited effect of endocrine therapy, the randomized comparison in clinical trials as a means of confirming hypotheses related to ways of improving treatment remains indispensable.

REFERENCES

1. Goldhirsch A, Gelber ED and Davis BW: Adjuvant chemotherapy trials in breast cancer: an appraisal and lessons for patient care outside the trials. In: JF Forbes (ed) Clinical Surgery International, Breast Disease 1986 (10) Chapter 10:123-138
2. UK BCTS, UICC, WHO: Review of mortality results in randomized trials in early breast cancer. Lancet 1984 (2):1205
3. Mouridsen H, Palshof T and Patterson J: Tamoxifen in advanced breast cancer. Cancer Treatment 1978 (5):131-141
4. Cole MP: A clinical trial of an artificial menopause in carcinoma of the breast. Inserm 1975 (55):143-150
5. Meakin JW, Allt WEC, Beale FA, Bush RS, Clark RM, Fitzpatrick PJ, Hawkins NV, Jenkin RDT, Pringle JF, Reid JG, Rider WD, Hayward JL and Bulbrook RD: Ovarian irradiation and prednisone following surgery and radiotherapy for carcinoma of the breast. Breast Cancer Res Treat 1983 (3):45-48
6. Bryant AJ and Weir JA: Prophylactic oophorectomy in operable instances of carcinoma of the breast. Surg Gynecol Obstet 1981 (153):660-664
7. Ludwig Breast Cancer Study Group: Chemotherapy with or without oophorectomy in high-risk premenopausal patients with operable breast cancer. J Clin Oncol 1985 (3):1059-1067
8. Bonadonna G, Rossi A, Valagussa P, Banfi A and Veronesi U: The CMF program for operable breast cancer with positive axillry nodes. Updated analysis on the disease-free interval, site of relapse and drug tolerance. Cancer 1977 (39):2904-2915
9. Goldhirsch A, for the Ludwig Breast Cancer Study Group: Adjuvant therapy for postmenopausal women with operable breast cancer. Part I, A randomized trial of chemo-endocrine vs. endocrine therapy vs. mastectomy alone. In: Jones SE and Salmon SE (eds) Adjuvant Therapy of Cancer 1984 (4):379-391 Orlando Grune & Stratton
10. Ludwig Breast Cancer Study Group: Randomized trial of chemo-endocrine therapy, endocrine therapy and mastectomy alone in postmenopausal patients with operable breast cancer and axillary node metastasis. Lancet 1984 (1):1256-1260
11. Taylor IV SG, Olsen JE, Cummings FJ and Knuiman M:

Observation compared to adjuvant chemo-hormonotherapy in postmenopausal breast cancer: the ECOG trial. Proc Am Soc Clin Oncol 1985 (4):61
12. Ludwig Breast Cancer Study Group: Adjuvant combination chemotherapy with or without prednisone in premenopausal breast cancer patients with metastases in 1 to 3 axillary lymph nodes: a randomized trial. Cancer Res 1985 (45):4454-4459
13. Brincker H, Mouridsen HT, Rank F, Rose C and Andersen KW: Evidence of a castration-medicated effect of adjuvant chemotherapy (CT) in a randomized trial of cyclophosphamide monotherapy versus CMF in premenopausal Stage II breast cancer. Proc Am Soc Clin Oncol 1985 (4):56
14. Rossi A, Bonadonna G, Tancini G, Bajetta E, Marchini S, Valagussa P and Veronesi U: Trials of adjuvant chemotherapy in breast cancer. The experience of the Istituto Nazionale Tumori of Milan. In: Mouridsen HT and Palshof T (eds) Breast cancer - experimental and clinical Aspects 1980: 149-156 Oxford: Pergamon Press
15. Fisher B, Sherman B, Rockette H, Redmond C, Margolese R and Fisher ER: l-Phenylalanine mustard (L-PAM) in the management of premenopausal patients with primary breast cancer: lack of association of DFS with depression of ovarian function. Cancer 1979 (44):847-857
16. Tormey DC: Clinical results III: Experience of randomized trials without surgical controls. In: Senn H (ed) Recent results in cancer research adjuvant chemotherapy of breast cancer. Heidelberg: Springer Verlag 1984: 155-165
17. Padmanabhan N, Howell A, Rubens RD: Adjuvant chemotherapy with cyclophosphamide, methotrexate and fluorouracil (CMF) in early breast cancer: mechanisms of action. Proc ASCO 1986 (5):59
18. Fisher B, Redmond C, Brown A: Adjuvant chemotherapy with and without tamoxifen in treatment of primary breast cancer: 5-year results from the National Surgical Adjuvant Breast and Bowel Project Trial. J Clin Oncol 1986 (4):459-471
19. Palshof T, Carstensen B, Briand P, Mouridsen HT and Dombernowsky P: Adjuvant endocrine therapy in . pre-and postmenopausal women with operable breast cancer. Rev Endocr Rel Cancer 1985 (17):43-51
20. Rose C, Mouridsen HT, Thorpe SM, Andersen J, Blichert-Toft M and Andersen for the Danish Breast Cancer Cooperative Group: Antiestrogen-treatment of postmenopausal women with primary high risk breast cancer. 72 months of life table analysis. Rev Endocr Rel Cancer 1985 (17):17-25
21. Wallgren A, Baral E, Nordenskjold B, Skoog L, Theve NO and Wilking N: Should adjuvant therapy be given for several years in breast cancer? In: Jones SE and Salmon SE (eds) Adjuvant therapy of cancer IV. Orlando: Grune & Stratton 1984: 331-337
22. Ribeiro G and Swindell R: The Christie Hospital tamoxifen (Nolvadex) adjuvant trial for operable breast carcinoma - 7 year results. Eur J Cancer Clin Oncol 1985 (21):897-900
23. Nolvadex Adjuvant Trial Organization: Controlled trial of tamoxifen as single adjuvant agent in management of early breast cancer: analysis at 6 years. Lancet 1985 (1):836-840
24. Pritchard KI, Meakin JW, Boyd NF, Ambus U, Dembo AJ, Evans WK, Sutherland DJA, Wilkinson RH, Bassett A, Campbell J and DeBoer G: A prospective randomized controlled trial of

adjuvant tamoxifen in postmenopausal women with axillary node-positive breast cancer. In: Jones SE and Salmon SE (eds) Adjuvant Therapy of Cancer IV. Orlando: Grune & Stratton 1984:339-347

25. Cummings FJ, Gray R, Davis TE, Tormey DC et al: Adjuvant tamoxifen therapy of elderly women with stage II breast cancer. Ann Int Med 1985 (103):324-329
26. Gelber RD for the Ludwig Breast Cancer Study Group: Adjuvant therapy for postmenopausal women with operable breast cancer: Part II - randomized trials comparing endocrine therapy with surgery alone. In: Jones SE and Salmon SE (eds) Adjuvant Therapy of Cancer IV. Orlando: Grune & Stratton 1984: 393-404
27. Hubay CA, Pearson OH, Marshall JS et al: Adjuvant therapy of Stage II breast cancer. Breast Cancer Res Treat 1981 (1):77-82
28. Rubins RD and Knight RK: The contribution of prednisolone (P) to primary endocrine therapy (PET) in primary breast cancer. Proc Am Soc Clin Oncol 1985 (4):53

Towards an Optimal Strategy for the Adjuvant Therapy of Breast Cancer.

V.C. Jordan

Departments of Human Oncology and Pharmacology, Wisconsin Clinical Cancer Center,
600 Highland Avenue, Madison, WI 53792, USA

The aim of adjuvant therapy, for node positive breast cancer patients following mastectomy, is to eradicate all of the micrometastatic lesions that are distributed around the body. In so doing, a cure can be achieved. Much of the clinical effort has focused upon chemotherapeutic regimens that have been shown to have success in the treatment of advanced disease. The theory which has dominated much of the thinking for the past decade is that the cell kill that can be achieved with a regimen in advanced disease should be capable of destroying a micrometastasis completely. Unfortunately, this has not been found to be the case, and interestingly enough, chemotherapy has only been found to be of significant value in premenopausal patients.

Antioestrogen therapy was adopted as a treatment strategy following the initiation of the early chemotherapeutic studies. It was argued that the lack of toxicity of an agent such as tamoxifen would allow daily treatment for at least a couple of years. Incorporation of tamoxifen into chemotherapeutic regimens, or its use alone as an adjuvant therapy has, in general, provided benefit for the patient (1,2,4,6,7,9,14,17, 21). The greatest benefit is, however, observed in postmenopausal patients who receive at least two years of tamoxifen treatment.

In this chapter, the endocrinology of adjuvant therapy in pre-and postmenopausal women will be considered in order to develop a rational strategy for the long-term survival of patients with node-positive breast cancer.

PREMENOPAUSAL PATIENTS

There are several types of adjuvant therapy that have been explored in clinical trial.

1) Chemotherapy

2) Tamoxifen

3) Chemotherapy plus tamoxifen

4) Chemotherapy plus continuous tamoxifen therapy

1. Chemotherapy

Adjuvant chemotherapy has achieved the most significant successes in premenopausal patients (3). This may be result of a chemosensitivity of rapidly growing disease in younger patients or an indirect effect of chemotherapy upon the endocrine system. Of course the final result could also be a combination of these actions.

Chemotherapy causes ovarian dysfunction, and continuous chemotherapy in patients over 40 years of age causes ovarian failure (19). In younger patients (30-40 years old) at least 12 months of chemotherapy may be required to cause ovarian failure. With this knowledge, it would be prudent to consider that ovarian ablation could account for the advantage observed for some premenopausal patients following adjuvant chemotherapy. At present, very little endocrinological research is focused upon resolving this hypothesis in current adjuvant trials. Retrospective evaluations of "amenorrhea" are inadequate to describe the endocrine changes that occur in a patient during the time following adjuvant therapy. If ovarian ablation is a factor in obtaining a response in the sensitive patients, then it would only be logical to ensure ovarian failure has occurred to prevent the tumour being activated by high circulating levels of the mitogen, oestradiol.

2. Tamoxifen

There are no large-scale trials that evaluate tamoxifen alone as an adjuvant therapy in premenopausal patients. There are, however, several trials that chose to include some premenopausal patients (1,2,17). It appears that these patients faired as well as their postmenopausal counterparts, but for the long term, this approach may not be the best overall strategy.

Tamoxifen is a competitive inhibitor of oestrogen binding in breast cancer cells (11). In the premenopausal patient, the antioestrogen causes a reflex rise in follicle-stimulating hormone which ultimately causes an increase in ovarian steroidogenesis. The circulating levels of oestrogen rise (20), which in turn can potentially overcome the competitive blockade by tamoxifen at the tumour oestrogen receptor. The fact that the blockade at the hypothalamopituitary axis is overcome by oestrogen to induce ovulation and maintain the menstrual cycle, speaks for the lack of efficiency of the antioestrogen.
It is possible that in the short term, tamoxifen is of benefit to prevent tumour cell replication (1-2 years), but in the long term, the increase in ovarian steroidogenesis will reverse tamoxifen's action.

3. Chemotherapy plus tamoxifen

The combination of tamoxifen plus chemotherapy brings together both of the concepts (increased steroidogenesis and ovarian failure) discussed for the individual strategies (18). Tamoxifen appears to maintain ovarian steroidogenesis so that at least 6-9 months of chemotherapy is required for ovarian ablation. This is

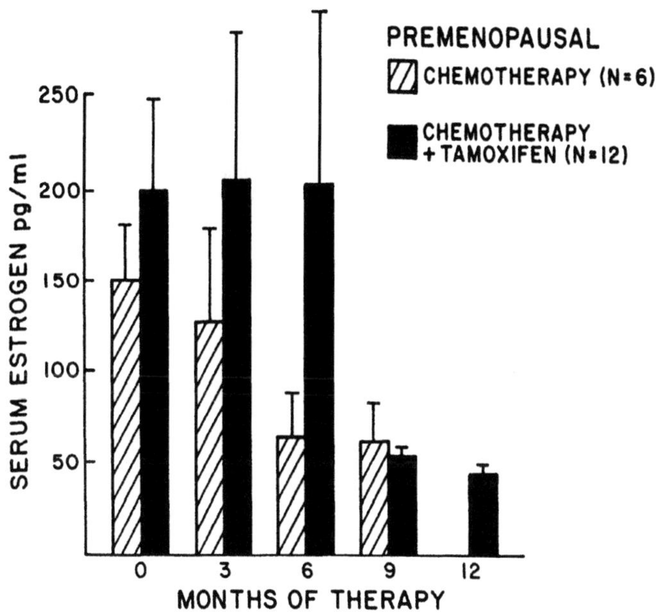

Figure 1. The decrease in circulating oestrogen (oestrone plus oestradiol) levels in premenopausal patients receiving either combination chemotherapy (CMF) or chemotherapy plus tamoxifen. Ovarian failure occurs between 6 and 9 months.

illustrated in Figure 1 where chemotherapy is compared with chemotherapy plus tamoxifen.

Although oestrogen levels (oestrogen and oestrone) are maintained for a longer period in patients treated with tamoxifen, this profile does not reflect the true picture. Tamoxifen causes very large individual increases in circulating oestrogens, but eventually ovarian failure occurs. The type of result that can be obtained is shown in the comparison of three patients receiving chemotherapy and three patients receiving chemotherapy plus tamoxifen (Figure 2).

The original rationale for combining tamoxifen and chemotherapy together appears to have been that tamoxifen would affect hormone-dependent cells in a heterogeneous tumour whereas chemotherapy would destroy hormone-independent cells. In general, a combination of tamoxifen and chemotherapy has not shown to be an advantage over chemotherapy alone and in fact in certain instances has been perceived to be a disadvantage. With the wisdom of hindsight, these results might have been predicted if chemotherapy is exerting an antihormonal effect after ovarian ablation and affecting the same cell population as the antioestrogen. Thus, the antioestrogen would not be expected to add too much more to the final result.

4. Chemotherapy plus long-term tamoxifen therapy

Short-term adjuvant chemotherapy requires the destruction of all breast cancer cells within a few weeks to cure the patient. This is the operating premise for this treatment strategy. The initial

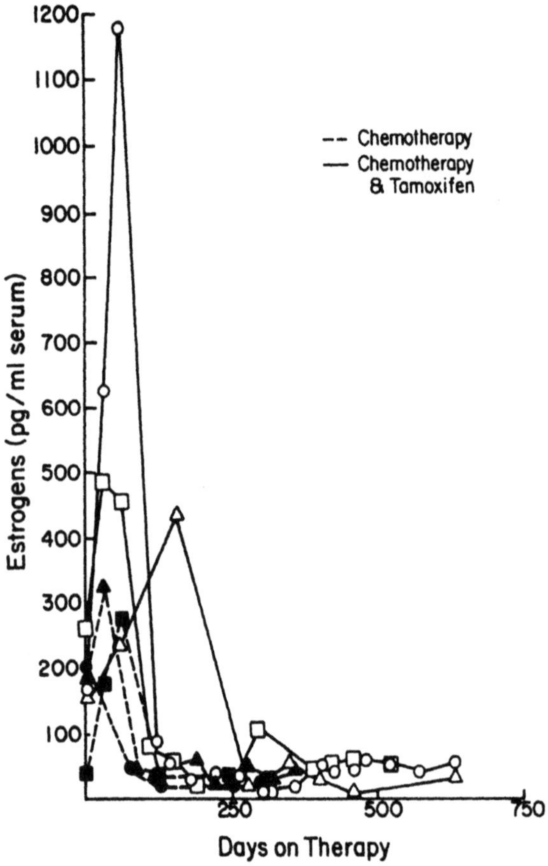

Figure 2. The early increase in circulating oestrogen (oestrone plus oestradiol) levels in premenopausal patients receiving tamoxifen with combination chemotherapy. Ovarian failure occurs after 9 months of therapy.

clinical experiments with one or two years of chemotherapy have been contracted to six months to produce the same clinical effect. It is perhaps not an accident that this is the time required for ovarian ablation. The other premise was that the action of the chemotherapy required no further considerations of environmental influences upon the tumour.

Even if chemotherapy exerts its primary effect through the ovary to produce an initial response to patients, adrenal steroids will ultimately act as a stimulus to provoke tumour regrowth. In fact, strategies of ovarian ablation followed by continuous administration of prednisone have yielded one of the most successful treatment approaches.

Clearly if successful ovarian ablation is achieved with chemotherapy, then continuous tamoxifen therapy, possibly for the lifetime of the patient, would be considered to be a viable alternative to avoid the side effects of glucocorticoids. In fact, this approach has been tried successfully at the University of Wisconsin Clinical Cancer Center (21). The tamoxifen therapy produces a blockade of oestrogen receptors to inhibit the mitogenic actions of circulating oestrogens. Adequate drug levels must, however, be maintained for prolonged periods because tamoxifen is a tumoristatic rather than tumoricidal agent. Therefore, for the strategy to be optimally effective, adequate drug levels must be present continuously in a low oestrogen environment.

One could imagine that this approach would be less than optimal in a high oestrogen environment. An increase in circulating oestrogens will reduce the efficiency of tamoxifen as a competitive inhibitor. This can occur in young women (<40 years old) who might be given a short course of chemotherapy (intensive regimens to minimize side effects) followed by continuous tamoxifen therapy. We have found that amenorrhoea occurs initially but, within a few months, ovulatory cycles resume. Oestrogen levels are elevated and the option of ovariectomy should be provided to regain the initiative in controlling occult disease.

POSTMENOPAUSAL PATIENTS

The same types of treatments that have been employed for premenopausal patients have been used for postmenopausal patients.

1) Chemotherapy

2) Tamoxifen

3) Chemotherapy plus tamoxifen

4) Chemotherapy plus continuous tamoxifen therapy

1. Chemotherapy

The first adjuvant study with L-phenylalanine mustard (5) in the United States demonstrated the potential value of adjuvant chemotherapy. Unfortunately, European experience has not produced the same optimistic results. Single or combination chemotherapy is not an advantage to postmenopausal women. Indeed, if chemotherapy exerts beneficial effects by ovarian ablation, then this approach would not be expected to be of value. However, combination chemotherapy plus prednisone has advantages over chemotherapy alone. It has been argued that the prednisone permits greater doses of chemotherapy to be administered. However, the adrenal suppressive effect of prednisone, and therefore the indirect endocrine effects are rarely addressed. Clearly, short-term (1-2 years) adrenal suppression (and ultimately the decrease in the production of androstenedione) would be expected to produce a short-term gain for the patient.

2. Tamoxifen

It is generally recognised that one to two years of adjuvant tamoxifen therapy can benefit postmenopausal patients who originally had estrogen receptor positive primary tumours. Combination of the clinical trials data has demonstrated benefit with tamoxifen, but as the drug is a tumoristatic rather than a tumoricidal agent, longer treatment schedules would be expected to be the most beneficial. The British NATO trial has claimed a survival advantage for patients following two years of treatment (2); however, longer treatments should be considered to produce the maximal benefit.

3. Chemotherapy plus tamoxifen

The addition of tamoxifen to combination chemotherapy regimens has been shown to provide benefit for the patients compared with chemotherapy alone (6). The most benefit is observed in those individuals with primary tumours that were oestrogen and progesterone receptor positive. However, termination of the tamoxifen at the end of chemotherapy results in an increase in the rate of recurrences. Again, this result would be expected for a drug with tumoristatic properties.

4. Chemotherapy plus continuous tamoxifen therapy

There are currently no firm data on the value of chemotherapy plus continuous tamoxifen therapy as an adjuvant in postmenopausal patients. However, the Eastern Cooperative Oncology Group is currently evaluating this approach in the protocol EST 5181. One year of chemotherapy (CMFPTH or alternating cycles of CMFPTH and $T^{s}AV^{b}TH$) is randomized to observation or continuous tamoxifen for a total of five years. Based upon experience at the University of Wisconsin Clinical Cancer Center (21), where tamoxifen is given indefinitely, as a third step, EST 5181 proposes to randomize to observation or continue tamoxifen indefinitely. These data should be available for evaluation by the end of the decade. Clearly though, extensive clinical experience has demonstrated that tamoxifen has a low incidence of side effects and is well tolerated for prolonged periods (8,21).

BACKGROUND AND RATIONALE FOR THE APPLICATION OF LONG-TERM ADJUVANT THERAPY WITH TAMOXIFEN IN A LOW OESTROGEN ENVIRONMENT

Tamoxifen is a tumoristatic agent upon breast cancer cells in culture (15), carcinogen-induced rat mammary carcinoma models (10,12,13) and breast cancer cells transplanted into athymic (nude) mice (16). Long treatment courses are the most effective at preventing cell replication and tumour growth, but when therapy is stopped, oestrogen can reactivate cell division. These principles, established in the laboratory, are currently being applied in clinical trial.

The mechanism of action of tamoxifen, almost certainly, involves the competitive blockade of oestrogen binding to the oestrogen receptor. Clearly therefore, tamoxifen will be the most effective in a low oestrogen environment. Chemotherapy may be beneficial in premenopausal patients by either a direct action on the tumour cells or indirectly by causing ovarian failure. Obviously, if the latter action is important, complete oophorectomy may be a viable, less troublesome alternative to the patient. Tamoxifen therapy in premenopausal patients may not be an optimal long-term strategy as increased steroidogenesis may ultimately cause tumour regrowth. Oophorectomy should be considered to avoid an increase in oestrogen levels.

Continuous tamoxifen therapy must be employed to maintain a blockade of tumour oestrogen receptors and prevent the direct action of steroids of adrenal origin or phyto-oestrogens from the diet. In this way, hormone-dependent cells may be prevented from replication, and delay the drift to hormone-independency. Obviously, the very nature of the sensitivity of the tumour cells to oestrogen makes the compliance of the patients and the bio-availability of the drug a primary concern to maintain the effectiveness of the therapy.

REFERENCES

1. Baum M and other members of the Nolvadex Adjuvant Trial Organization. Controlled trial of tamoxifen as adjuvant agent in management of early breast cancer. Lancet 1983 (1):257-261
2. Baum M and other members of the Nolvadex Adjuvant Trial Orgazination. Controlled trial of tamoxifen as single adjuvant agent in management of early cancer. Lancet 1985 (1):836-840
3. Bonadonna G, Rossi A, Tancini G, Brambilla C and Valagussa P: Adjuvant chemotherapy trials in resectable breast cancer with positive axillary nodes. The experience of the Milan Cancer Institute. In: SE Jones and Salmon E (eds) Adjuvant Therapy of Cancer 1984 (4):195 New York: Grune and Stratton
4. Cummings FJ, Gray R, David TE, Tormey DC, Harris JE, Falkson G and Arseneau J: Adjuvant tamoxifen treatment of elderly women with stage II breast cancer. A double-blind comparison with placebo. Ann Int Med 1985 (103):324-329
5. Fisher B, Carbone PP, Econamou SG, Frelick R, Glass A, Lerner H, Redmond C, Zelen M, Band P, Katarych DL, Wolmark N and Fisher ER: L-phenylalanine mustard (L-PAM) in the management of primary breast cancer: a report of early findings. N Engl J Med 1975 (292):117-122
6. Fisher B, Redmond C, Brown A, Wickerman DL, Wolmark N, Allergra J, Escher G, Lippmann M, Savlov E, Wittliff JL and Fisher ER: Influence of tumor estrogen and progesterone receptor levels on the response to tamoxifen and chemotherapy in primary breast cancer. J Clin Oncol 1983 (1): 227-241
7. Fisher B, Redmond C, Wolmark N, Wittliff JL, Fisher ER, PLotkin D, Bowman D, Sachs S, Wolter J, Frelich R, Desser R, DiCalzi N, Geggie P, Campell T, Elias EG, Prayer D, Koontz P, Volk TT, Dimitrov N, Gardner B, Lerner H, Shibata H and other NSABP investigators: Treatment of primary breast cancer with chemotherapy and tamoxifen. N Engl J Med 1981 (305):1-6
8. Furr BJA and Jordan VC: The pharmacology and clinical uses of tamoxifen. Pharmac & Ther 1984 (25):127-205

9. Hubay CA, Pearson OH, Marshall JS, Rhodes RS, DeBame SM, Rosenblatt J, Mansour EG, Herman RE, Jones JC, Flynn WJ, Eckert C, McGuire Wl and 27 participating investigators: Adjuvant chemotherapy antioestrogen therapy and immunotherapy for stage II breast cancer. Cancer 1980 (46):2805-2808
10. Jordan VC: Use of the DMBA-induced rat mammary carcinoma system for the evaluation of tamoxifen as a potential adjuvant therapy. Rev on Endocr Related Cancer (October supplement) 1978 : 49-55
11. Jordan VC: The biochemical pharmacology of antiestrogen action. Pharm Rev 1984 (36):245-276
12. Jordan VC, Dix CJ and Allen KE: The effectiveness of long-term tamoxifen treatment in a laboratory model for adjuvant hormone therapy of breast cancer. In: Salmon SE and Jones JE (eds) Adjuvant Therapy of Cancer 1979 (2):19-26 New York: Grune & Stratton Inc
13. Jordan VC, Mirecki DM and Gottardis MM: Continuous tamoxifen treatment prevents the appearance of mammary tumors in a model of adjuvant therapy. In: Jones SE and Salmon SE (eds) Adjuvant Therapy of Cancer 1984 (4):27-33 New York: Grune & Stratton Inc
14. Ludwig Breast Cancer Study Group. Randomized trial of chemoendocrine therapy, endocrine therapy and mastectomy alone in postmenopausal patients with operable breast cancer and axillary node metastases. Lancet 1984 (1):1256-1260
15. Osborne CK, Boldt DH, Clark GM and Trent JML: Effects of tamoxifen on human breast cancer cell cycle kinetics: accumulation of cells in early G1 phase. Cancer Res 1983 (43):3583-3585
16. Osborne CK, Hobbs K and Clark GM: Effect of estrogen and antiestrogens on growth of human breast cancer cells in athymic nude mice. Cancer Res 1985 (45):584-590
17. Ribeiro G and Swindell R: The Christie Hospital tamoxifen (Nolvadex) adjuvant trial for operable breast carcinoma: seven-year results. Eur J Cancer Clin Oncol 1985 (21):897-900
18. Rose DP and Davis TE: Effects of adjuvant chemohormonaltherapy on the ovarian and adrenal function of breast cancer patients. Cancer Res 1983 (40):4043-4047
19. Rose DP and Davis TE: Ovarian function in patients receiving adjuvant chemotherapy for breast cancer. Lancet 1977 (1):1174-1176
20. Sherman BM, Chapler FK, Crickard K and Wycoff D: Endcorine consequences of continuous antiestrogen therapy with tamoxifen in premenopausal women. J Clin Invest 1979 (64): 398-404
21. Tormey DC and Jordan VC: Long-term tamoxifen adjuvant therapy in node positive breast cancer: a metabolic and pilot clinical study. Breast Cancer Res Treat 1984 (4):297-302

Tamoxifen Prophylaxis: Prevention is Better Than Cure – Prevention is Cure?

V. C. Jordan

Departments of Human Oncology and Pharmacology, Wisconsin Clinical Cancer Center, 600 Highland Avenue, Madison, WI 53792, USA

The treatment of advanced breast cancer with surgery, hormonal modalities, radiotherapy and chemotherapy has met with palliation in the face of relentlessy progressive disease. The remarkable successes observed with chemotherapy in testicular carcinoma, Hodgkin's disease or childhood leukaemias are rarely, if ever, observed in advanced breast cancer. Often the gains made are at a price. Discomfort and side effects are the patients' constant companions during rigorous chemotherapy regimens. Unfortunately, objective and complete responses invariably turn to rapidly growing drug-and radiation-resistant disease.

Strategies in the 1970s to treat minimal (node positive) disease with chemotherapy following mastectomy were based upon the fact that, to cure patients, all tumour cells must be eradicated. The ability of chemotherapy to achieve this is dependent upon initial tumour mass. Thus, with minimal tumour mass, adjuvant chemotherapy was projected to have a favourable chance at success. Unfortunately, initial trials have not met with anything like uniform success. The reasons for this are complex but may reflect our ignorance about the cell kinetics of minimal breast cancer (i.e., small clusters of metastatic tumour cells may lie dormant in a nutritionally deprived environment, not unlike spores in relation to bacteria, and as such are resistant to chemotherapy). Alternatively, less rigorous chemotherapeutic regimens are used compared to the best aggressive approaches in advanced disease.

Most success at delaying disease recurrence has been achieved with 1) antioestrogenic therapy in post menopausal patients and 2) combination chemotherapy regimens in premenopausal patients. Both therapeutic regimens could be described as "antihormonal" approaches, i.e., 1) blocking oestrogen action in the tumour and 2) causing a sharp decrease in ovarian steroids by ovarian failure.

These clues to the successful application of agents for the therapy of breast cancer suggest that an effective chemopreventive agent might have a chance at controlling the few malingnant cells. The aim of this chapter is to consider the potential application of antioestrogens for the chemoprevention of breast cancer.

Obviously certain definitions and limitations to this approach to breast cancer therapy must be stated at the outset.

Chemoprevention, as the name implies, requires the agent to prevent the initiation and perhaps the promotional aspects in the development of breast cancer. Tamoxifen prevents the initiation and promotion (4) of carcinogen-induced rat mammary cancer; success in maintaining the rat tumour free is proportional to the length of treatment from the carcinogenic insult (5). In humans, the experiment is less readily undertaken as the precise time (or even identification) of the carcinogenic insult is unknown. Even if the time of the insult were known, the administrative and toxicological problems of treating, for example, a population of teenagers for 10 years may be too overwhelming to consider. Therefore, all current proposals to treat populations with antioestrogens must be considered to be <u>chemosuppressive</u> approaches, i.e., occult hormone-dependent tumour cells will be held in a state of suspended animation as long as the therapy is continued. The length of therapy may be important in preventing tumour development but may, in of as itself, be unable to reverse tumorigenesis. In this regard, the immune system of the patients may be of prime importance if cures are to be secured. An active immune system might be able to neutralise a clone of static tumour cells but unable to respond to an expanding population. No evidence for this action of the immune system has been demonstrated for breast cancer; however, the benign actions of tamoxifen when compared to chemotherapy will permit immunological anticancer mechanisms to occur if they do indeed exist.

Clearly the incidence of breast cancer is too low to undertake a chemosuppressive trial with tamoxifen upon breast cancer incidence in "high risk" groups, for example, women who have had a mother and a sister with breast cancer. Additionally, women with low circulating levels of sex hormone binding globulin or a history of benign breast disease would be potential target populations (2).

The time at which to undertake a clinical chemosuppressive trial with an antioestrogen is very important. Obviously, if there is hope of complete cure (prevention?) for the patient, the courses of drug could be given to younger women in order to gain maximal benefit for all women. Unfortunately, there is very little evidence to support the position that antioestrogens can reverse the process of tumorigenesis. Thus, long-term (5-10 years) therapy of premenopausal patients is required <u>to delay</u> the appearance of occult tumours.

Since tamoxifen is an antioestrogen, then the thesis requires the drug to prevent the promotion or progression of the hormone-dependent disease by competitively blocking the oestrogen receptor. However, the antioestrogen will also create an inhibition of the negative feedback system of oestrogen from the ovary to the hypothalamo-pituitary axis. As a result, the antioestrogen would be expected to increase the output of gonadotrophins, mainly follicle-stimulating hormone.
Oestrogen levels do increase in premenopausal patients following short courses of tamoxifen (3,6), but as yet there are no reports about the impact of many years of tamoxifen treatment on the endocrine system. Clearly, if oestrogen levels increase in order to overcome the antioestrogen blockade at the hypothalamo-pituitary axis, there is little likelihood that

tamoxifen can produce indefinite antioestrogen effects in the occult tumour.

The impact of tamoxifen on the endocrine system raises a broader issue of potential side effects to a majority of individuals who will not experience breast cancer. Large populations of women will be at risk of pregnancy and decisions of contraception or abortion will be required. There is little information about the potential teratogenicity of tamoxifen in animal systems and, as yet, no studies have been completed in primates.

Ovarian failure at the time of menopause is considered to be a major factor in the subsequent development of osteoporosis in postmenopausal women. Whether the administration of antioestrogen to premenopausal women will result in an early onset of osteoporosis remains to be determined. It is possible that the actions of oestrogen on proliferative tissue are different than those on bone and calcium mobilisation. In fact, the partial oestrogenic activity of tamoxifen may be supportive rather than deleterious in this instance.

These potential toxicological considerations in premenopausal women could be avoided by the study of postmenopausal women. This also has the advantage of being at a time of increasing tumour occurrence (50-70 years of age). A trial incorporating large patient numbers (10,000+) to treatment (5-10 years) or placebos would be expected to produce the greatest differences in a chemosuppressive study. If this strategy is developed, the principal toxicological problems will focus upon osteoporosis and the development of thromboembolic disorders. Study of the osteoporosis question should be initiated as soon as possible to determine the immediate impact (1 year) of tamoxifen therapy upon bone density. There have been isolated reports about the incidence of thromboembolic disease associated with tamoxifen therapy. However, these are rarely associated with the administration of tamoxifen alone. Tamoxifen does decrease antithrombin III levels in patients with advanced breast cancer, but this is, in general, not of clinical significance. Nevertheless, patients with a history of thromboembolic disorders should not be admitted to chemosuppressive studies.

Finally, there is little known about the long-term effects of tamoxifen upon the postmenopausal uterus. Tamoxifen produces oestrogen-like effects but continued stimulation may have deleterious effects upon this organ. Furthermore, the antioestrogenic effects observed in breast tissue may not be reflected in occult endometrial carcinoma. While tamoxifen has been successfully employed to control the growth of metastatic disease, no studies have been conducted upon the primary tumour. A recent report of a hormone-dependent human carcinoma cell line grown in athymic mice has demonstrated that tamoxifen can support tumour growth (1). Clearly, clinicians must remain vigilant to the possibility of an increased occurrence of uterine carcinoma.

In summary, there are currently many proposals to use tamoxifen as a chemosuppressive agent, but it should be clear from the foregoing arguments that the drug should only be used under specific circumstances and with adequate safeguards. Well-controlled clinical studies with effective patient monitoring must be undertaken to prevent the inappropriate application of an innovative drug with few toxicological problems. Only in this way can an adequate evaluation of this approach to breast cancer treatment be made.

REFERENCES

1. Clark CL and Satyaswaroop PG: Photoaffinity labeling of the progesterone receptor from human endometrial carcinoma. Cancer Res 1985 (45):5417-5420
2. Cuzick J, Wang DY and Bulbrook RD: The prevention of breast cancer. Lancet 1986 (1):83-86
3. Groom GV and Griffiths K: Effect of the antioestrogen tamoxifen on plasma levels of luteinizing hormone, follicle stimulating hormone, prolactin, and oestradiol and progesterone in normal pre-menopausal women. J Endocrinology 1976 (70):421-428
4. Jordan VC: Effect of tamoxifen (ICI 46,47) on initn and growth of DMBA-induced rat mammary carcinomata. Europ J Cancer 1976 (12):419-424
5. Jordan VC: Laboratory studies to develop general principles for the adjuvant treatment of breast cancer with antioestrogen: problems and potential for future clinical applications. Breast Cancer Res Treat 1983 (3) :73-86
6. Sherman BM, Chapler F, Crickard K and Wycoff D: Endocrine consequences of continuous antiestrogen therapy with tamoxifen in premenopausal women. J Clin Invest 1979 (64):318-404

MIX
Papier aus verantwortungsvollen Quellen
Paper from responsible sources
FSC® C105338

If you have any concerns about our products,
you can contact us on
ProductSafety@springernature.com

In case Publisher is established outside the EU,
the EU authorized representative is:
Springer Nature Customer Service Center GmbH
Europaplatz 3, 69115 Heidelberg, Germany

Printed by Libri Plureos GmbH
in Hamburg, Germany